Travel and Adventure Medicine

Editors

PAUL S. POTTINGER
CHRISTOPHER A. SANFORD

MEDICAL CLINICS OF NORTH AMERICA

www.medical.theclinics.com

Consulting Editors
DOUGLAS S. PAAUW
EDWARD R. BOLLARD

March 2016 • Volume 100 • Number 2

ELSEVIER

1600 John F. Kennedy Boulevard • Suite 1800 • Philadelphia, Pennsylvania, 19103-2899

http://www.theclinics.com

MEDICAL CLINICS OF NORTH AMERICA Volume 100, Number 2
March 2016 ISSN 0025-7125, ISBN-13: 978-0-323-41651-1

Editor: Jessica McCool
Developmental Editor: Alison Swety

Medical Clinics of North America (ISSN 0025-7125) is published bimonthly by Elsevier Inc., 360 Park Avenue South, New York, NY 10010-1710. Months of publication are January, March, May, July, September, and November. Business and editorial offices: 1600 John F. Kennedy Boulevard, Suite 1800, Philadelphia, PA 19103-2899. Periodicals postage paid at New York, NY, and additional mailing offices. Subscription prices are USD $260.00 per year (US individuals), $531.00 per year (US institutions), $100.00 per year (US Students), $320.00 per year (Canadian individuals), $690.00 per year (Canadian institutions), $200.00 per year (Canadian and foreign students), $390.00 per year (foreign individuals), and $690.00 per year (foreign institutions). To receive student/resident rate, orders must be accompanied by name of affiliated institution, date of term, and the signature of program/residency coordinator on institution letterhead. Orders will be billed at individual rate until proof of status is received. Foreign air speed delivery is included in all Clinics' subscription prices. All prices are subject to change without notice. **POSTMASTER:** Send address changes to *Medical Clinics of North America*, Elsevier Health Sciences Division, Subscription Customer Service, 3251 Riverport Lane, Maryland Heights, MO 63043. **Customer Service: Telephone: 1-800-654-2452** (U.S. and Canada); **1-314-447-8871** (outside U.S. and Canada). **Fax: 314-447-8029. E-mail: journalscustomerserviceusa@elsevier.com** (for print support); **journalsonlinesupport-usa@elsevier.com** (for online support).

Reprints. For copies of 100 or more of articles in this publication, please contact the Commercial Reprints Department, Elsevier Inc., 360 Park Avenue South, New York, NY 10010-1710. Tel.: 212-633-3874; Fax: 212-633-3820; E-mail: reprints@elsevier.com.

Medical Clinics of North America is also published in Spanish by McGraw-Hill Interamericana Editores S. A., P.O. Box 5-237, 06500 Mexico, D.F., Mexico.

Medical Clinics of North America is covered in *MEDLINE/PubMed (Index Medicus), Current Contents, ASCA, Excerpta Medica, Science Citation Index, and ISI/BIOMED.*

PROGRAM OBJECTIVE

The goal of the *Medical Clinics of North America* is to keep practicing physicians up to date with current clinical practice by providing timely articles reviewing the state of the art in patient care.

TARGET AUDIENCE

All practicing physicians and other healthcare professionals.

LEARNING OBJECTIVES

Upon completion of this activity, participants will be able to:

1. Review common illnesses and injuries to people traveling in developing countries.
2. Discuss important immunizations and other personal protection measures for travellers.
3. Recognize the essentials of adventure, wilderness, and extreme sports medicine.

ACCREDITATION

The Elsevier Office of Continuing Medical Education (EOCME) is accredited by the Accreditation Council for Continuing Medical Education (ACCME) to provide continuing medical education for physicians.

The EOCME designates this enduring material for a maximum of 15 *AMA PRA Category 1 Credit*(s)™. Physicians should claim only the credit commensurate with the extent of their participation in the activity.

All other health care professionals requesting continuing education credit for this enduring material will be issued a certificate of participation.

DISCLOSURE OF CONFLICTS OF INTEREST

The EOCME assesses conflict of interest with its instructors, faculty, planners, and other individuals who are in a position to control the content of CME activities. All relevant conflicts of interest that are identified are thoroughly vetted by EOCME for fair balance, scientific objectivity, and patient care recommendations. EOCME is committed to providing its learners with CME activities that promote improvements or quality in healthcare and not a specific proprietary business or a commercial interest.

The planning committee, staff, authors and editors listed below have identified no financial relationships or relationships to products or devices they or their spouse/life partner have with commercial interest related to the content of this CME activity:

Francis Afukaar, MSc; Whitney Alexander, MD; Jonathan D. Alpern, MD; David R. Boulware, MD, MPH, CTropMed; Steven Bright, MD; Patrick Burns, MD; Pham Viet Cuong, PhD; Benjamin J. Dolan, MD; Stephen J. Dunlop, MD, MPH, CTropMed, FACEP; Anjali Fortna; Claire Fung, MD, MPH; Stanley L. Giddings, MD; Andrew Thomas Gomez, MD; William O. Hahn, MD; Nicholas J. Johnson, MD; David Mitchell Kanze, DO; Sharon Brown Kunin, DO, MS; Daniel T. Leung, MD, MSc; Andrew M. Luks, MD; Jessica McCool; Martha C. Hijar Medina, PhD; Charles Mock, MD, PhD, FACS; Kristian R. Olson, MD, MPH, DTM&H; Douglas S. Paauw, MD, MACP; Paul S. Pottinger, MD, DTM&H, FIDSA; Santha Priya; Ashwin Rao, MD; Christopher A. Sanford, MD, MPH, DTM&H; William M. Stauffer, MD, MSPH, FASTMH; Barclay T. Stewart, MD, MScPH; Geren S. Stone, MD, DTM&H; Megan Suermann; Anne C. Terry, RN, MSN, ARNP; David Townes, MD, MPH, DTM&H; Isaac Kofi Yankson, MPH.

The planning committee, staff, authors and editors listed below have identified financial relationships or relationships to products or devices they or their spouse/life partner have with commercial interest related to the content of this CME activity:

N. Jean Haulman, MD, MPH is on the speakers' bureau for, and a consultant/advisor for, Sanofi Pasteur SA.

Elaine C. Jong, MD, FIDSA, FASTMH is a consultant/advisor for Valneva SE, and receives royalties/patents from Elsevier B.V.

A. Michal Stevens, MD, MPH has stock ownership in Chimerix.

UNAPPROVED/OFF-LABEL USE DISCLOSURE

The EOCME requires CME faculty to disclose to the participants:

1. When products or procedures being discussed are off-label, unlabelled, experimental, and/or investigational (not US Food and Drug Administration [FDA] approved); and
2. Any limitations on the information presented, such as data that are preliminary or that represent ongoing research, interim analyses, and/or unsupported opinions. Faculty may discuss information about pharmaceutical agents that is outside of FDA-approved labelling. This information is intended solely for CME and is not intended to promote off-label use of these medications. If you have any questions, contact the medical affairs department of the manufacturer for the most recent prescribing information.

TO ENROLL

To enroll in the *Medical Clinics of North America* Continuing Medical Education program, call customer service at 1-800-654-2452 or sign up online at http://www.theclinics.com/home/cme. The CME program is available to subscribers for an additional annual fee of USD $295.

METHOD OF PARTICIPATION

In order to claim credit, participants must complete the following:

1. Complete enrolment as indicated above.
2. Read the activity.
3. Complete the CME Test and Evaluation. Participants must achieve a score of 70% on the test. All CME Tests and Evaluations must be completed online.

CME INQUIRIES/SPECIAL NEEDS

For all CME inquiries or special needs, please contact elsevierCME@elsevier.com.

MEDICAL CLINICS OF NORTH AMERICA

FORTHCOMING ISSUES

May 2016
Medical Care for Kidney and Liver Transplant Recipients
David A. Sass and
Alden M. Doyle, *Editors*

July 2016
Pharmacologic Therapy
Douglas S. Paauw and Kim O'Connor, *Editors*

September 2016
Quality Patient Care: Making Evidence-Based, High Value Choices
Marc Shalaby and Edward R. Bollard, *Editors*

RECENT ISSUES

January 2016
Managing Chronic Pain
Charles E. Argoff, *Editor*

November 2015
Dermatology
Roy M. Colven, *Editor*

September 2015
Comprehensive Care of the Patient with Chronic Illness
Douglas S. Paauw, *Editor*

RELATED INTEREST

Infectious Disease Clinics of North America, March 2015 (Vol. 29, Issue 1)
***Clostridium difficile* Infection**
Mark H. Wilcox, *Editor*
http://www.id.theclinics.com/

Contributors

CONSULTING EDITORS

DOUGLAS S. PAAUW, MD, MACP
Professor of Medicine, Division of General Internal Medicine, Rathmann Family Foundation Endowed Chair for Patient-Centered Clinical Education; Medicine Student Programs, Professor of Medicine, University of Washington School of Medicine, Seattle, Washington

EDWARD R. BOLLARD, MD, DDS, FACP
Professor of Medicine, Associate Dean of Graduate Medical Education, Designated Institutional Official, Department of Medicine, Penn State-Hershey Medical Center, Penn State University College of Medicine, Hershey, Pennsylvania

EDITORS

PAUL S. POTTINGER, MD, DTM&H, FIDSA
Associate Professor, Division of Allergy and Infectious Diseases, Department of Medicine, University of Washington, Seattle, Washington

CHRISTOPHER A. SANFORD, MD, MPH, DTM&H
Associate Professor, Family Medicine, Associate Professor, Global Health, University of Washington, Seattle, Washington

AUTHORS

FRANCIS AFUKAAR, MSc
Chief Research Scientist, Building and Road Research Institute, Kumasi, Ghana

WHITNEY ALEXANDER, MD
Resident Physician, Division of Emergency Medicine, University of Washington School of Medicine, Seattle, Washington

JONATHAN D. ALPERN, MD
Infectious Disease Fellow, University of Minnesota, Minneapolis, Minnesota

DAVID R. BOULWARE, MD, MPH, CTropMed
Lois and Richard King Distinguished Associate Professor, Infectious Disease and International Medicine, Department of Medicine, University of Minnesota, Minneapolis, Minnesota

STEVEN BRIGHT, MD
Resident Physician, Division of Emergency Medicine, University of Washington School of Medicine, Seattle, Washington

PATRICK BURNS, MD
Resident Physician, Division of Emergency Medicine, University of Washington School of Medicine, Seattle, Washington

PHAM VIET CUONG, PhD
Director, Center for Injury Policy and Prevention Research; Head, Department of Public Health Informatics, Hanoi School of Public Health, Hanoi, Vietnam

BENJAMIN J. DOLAN, MD
Emergency Medicine Resident, Hennepin County Medical Center, Minneapolis, Minnesota

STEPHEN J. DUNLOP, MD, MPH, CTropMed, FACEP
Assistant Professor of Emergency Medicine, Departments of Emergency Medicine and Medicine, Hennepin County Medical Center, University of Minnesota, Minneapolis, Minnesota

CLAIRE FUNG, MD, MPH
Family Physician, The Everett Clinic at Snohomish, Snohomish; Clinical Instructor, Department of Family Medicine, University of Washington Family Medicine Residency, Seattle, Washington

STANLEY L. GIDDINGS, MD
Division of Infectious Diseases, Department of Medicine, University of Utah School of Medicine, Salt Lake City, Utah

ANDREW THOMAS GOMEZ, MD
Resident Physician, Family Medicine, University of Washington, Seattle, Washington

WILLIAM O. HAHN, MD
Fellow, Division of Allergy and Infectious Diseases, Department of Medicine, University of Washington, Seattle, Washington

N. JEAN HAULMAN, MD, MPH
Assistant Clinical Faculty, Department of Pediatrics; Board Certification Pediatrics, Emergency Medicine, ISTM Certification in Travel Medicine, Exam Completion ASTMH, Vaccine Speaker for Sanofi Pasteur, University of Washington, Seattle, Washington

NICHOLAS J. JOHNSON, MD
Senior Fellow, Critical Care Medicine, Division of Pulmonary and Critical Care Medicine, Harborview Medical Center, University of Washington, Seattle, Washington

ELAINE C. JONG, MD, FIDSA, FASTMH
Division of Allergy and Infectious Diseases, Clinical Professor Emeritus, Department of Medicine, University of Washington, Seattle, Washington

DAVID MITCHELL KANZE, DO
Interim Director of Medical Education, Director, Family Medicine/Osteopathic Manipulative Treatment Residency Program, Skagit Regional Health, Mount Vernon, Washington

SHARON BROWN KUNIN, DO, MS
Global Health Fellow, Department of Family Medicine, University of Washington, Seattle, Washington

DANIEL T. LEUNG, MD, MSc
Division of Infectious Diseases, Department of Medicine; Division of Microbiology and Immunology, Department of Pathology, University of Utah School of Medicine, Salt Lake City, Utah

ANDREW M. LUKS, MD
Associate Professor of Medicine, Division of Pulmonary and Critical Care Medicine, Harborview Medical Center, University of Washington, Seattle, Washington

MARTHA C. HIJAR MEDINA, PhD
Secretaria Técnica del Consejo Nacional para la Prevención de Accidentes, Subsecretaría de Prevención y Promoción de la Salud, Ministry of Health, Mexico DF, Mexico

CHARLES MOCK, MD, PhD, FACS
Professor, Departments of Surgery, Epidemiology and Global Health, University of Washington; Harborview Injury Prevention and Research Center, Harborview Medical Center, Seattle, Washington

KRISTIAN R. OLSON, MD, MPH, DTM&H
Department of Medicine, MGH Center for Global Health, CAMTech Medical Director, Massachusetts General Hospital, Boston, Massachusetts

PAUL S. POTTINGER, MD, DTM&H, FIDSA
Associate Professor, Division of Allergy and Infectious Diseases, Department of Medicine, University of Washington, Seattle, Washington

ASHWIN RAO, MD
Program Director, Primary Care Sports Medicine Fellowship, Sports Medicine Section; Associate Professor, Family Medicine, University of Washington, Seattle, Washington

CHRISTOPHER A. SANFORD, MD, MPH, DTM&H
Associate Professor, Family Medicine, Associate Professor, Global Health, University of Washington, Seattle, Washington

WILLIAM M. STAUFFER, MD, MSPH, FASTMH
Professor, Division of Infectious Diseases and International Medicine, Department of Medicine, University of Minnesota, Minneapolis, Minnesota

A. MICHAL STEVENS, MD, MPH
Division of Infectious Diseases, Department of Medicine, University of Utah School of Medicine, Salt Lake City, Utah

BARCLAY T. STEWART, MD, MScPH
NIH/Fogarty Global Health Fellow, Department of Surgery, University of Washington, Seattle, Washington; School of Medical Sciences, Kwame Nkrumah University of Science and Technology, Kumasi, Ghana; Department of Surgery, Komfo Anokye Teaching Hospital, Kumasi, Ghana

GEREN S. STONE, MD, DTM&H
Department of Medicine, MGH Center for Global Health, Global Primary Care Program Director, Massachusetts General Hospital, Boston, Massachusetts

ANNE C. TERRY, RN, MSN, ARNP
Manager, UW Medicine Travel Clinic at Hall Health Center; Certificate in Infectious Disease, Certificate in Travel Health-International Society of Travel Medicine, University of Washington, Seattle, Washington

DAVID TOWNES, MD, MPH, DTM&H
Division of Emergency Medicine, Department of Global Health, University of Washington School of Medicine, Seattle, Washington

ISAAC KOFI YANKSON, MPH
Scientific Officer, Building and Road Research Institute, Kumasi, Ghana

Contents

Foreword

Travel and Adventure Medicine

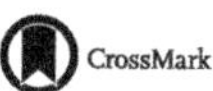

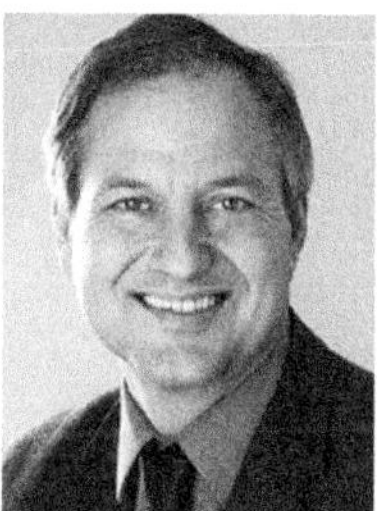

Douglas S. Paauw, MD, MACP
Consulting Editor

About 30 million US citizens travel outside the North America continent annually. Physicians are asked to provide pretravel advice and posttravel care for many of these travelers. In the past few decades, the popularity of wilderness and high-altitude exploration and extreme sporting activities has grown. This issue of *Medical Clinics of North America* devoted to travel and adventure medicine reviews important topics to help health care providers care for these patients as well as help prepare health care workers for their own travels and adventures. Paul S. Pottinger and Christopher A. Sanford have done an outstanding job bringing together a diverse set of topics. More traditional travel medicine concerns, such as malaria prevention, immunization, traveler's diarrhea, and treatment of the returning international traveler, are covered with timely up-to-date information. Articles covering the ethics of volunteerism, the travel medical kit, and road traffic injuries in travelers in developing countries are excellent additions to round out the travel medicine portion of this issue. A diverse set of adventure medicine topics, including high-altitude and wilderness medicine as well as an article on adventure and extreme sports, touches on a wide range of areas that is not frequently covered. I know you will find this a valuable and enjoyable issue.

Douglas S. Paauw, MD, MACP
Division of General Internal Medicine
Department of Medicine
University of Washington School of Medicine
Seattle, WA 98195, USA

E-mail address:
DPaauw@medicine.washington.edu

Med Clin N Am 100 (2016) xv
http://dx.doi.org/10.1016/j.mcna.2015.11.003

Preface

Travel and Adventure Medicine

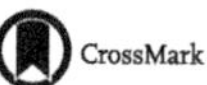

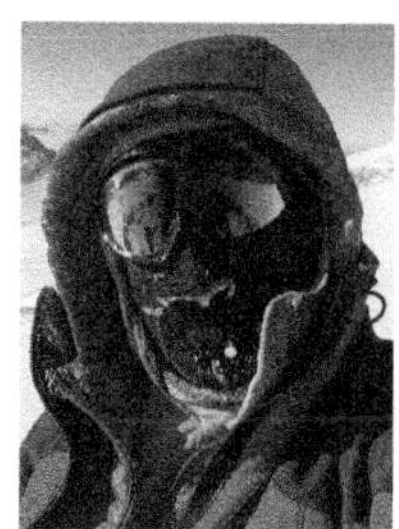

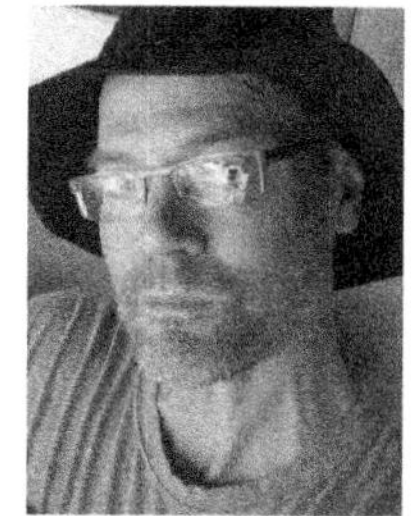

Paul S. Pottinger, MD, DTM&H, FIDSA   Christopher A. Sanford, MD, MPH, DTM&H
Editors

When your humble editors were in high school, adventurous kids traveled to France for a semester. Now it is routine for students—from elementary school to college—to visit remote and rustic destinations in low-income nations in South America, Africa, Asia, and elsewhere. International travel is on the increase to unprecedented levels, across the board, among tourists, athletes, volunteers, and those on business.

Medical providers who provide pretravel and/or posttravel care must familiarize themselves with common threats to international travelers to low-income nations as well as common illnesses seen in illreturned travelers. Caring for those who reside in a high-income nation does not prepare us to care for travelers to low-income destinations: both infectious and noninfectious problems may differ significantly from those encountered in wealthier regions of North America. The regular appearance of new infectious threats is the rule rather than the exception, and vaccine indications and schedules are forever changing. Thus, pretravel medicine providers are obligatorily students for life.

In former times, pretravel care consisted of receiving some immunizations, malaria prophylaxis, and little else. And while pretravel vaccinations and malaria prophylaxis are important components of the pretravel consultation, we now know that the greatest threats to international travelers are noninfectious; they include traffic injuries and drowning. Taking into account a traveler's personal medical history, itinerary, and planned activities, the pretravel provider can reduce the risk from threats as disparate as influenza and motorcycle crashes.

A panoply of new sports, from flying in wingsuits to zorbing, has arisen in recent years. Research on the health implications of these nascent sports is scant but rapidly accumulating. It is our hope that this collection of articles will help pretravel and posttravel medical providers provide state-of-the-art care to their travelers.

A wide range of travelers—from newborns to the elderly, from Iron Man triathletes to those debilitated with chronic illnesses—are traveling to increasingly remote destinations. Given that medical care in most low-income nations lags behind that practiced

Med Clin N Am 100 (2016) xvii–xviii
http://dx.doi.org/10.1016/j.mcna.2015.11.002
medical.theclinics.com
0025-7125/16/$ – see front matter

in high-income nations, it is important to minimize the odds of illness and injury while abroad and counsel travelers regarding self-treatment and accessing appropriate medical care should a mishap occur.

Many travelers recall their time overseas as high points of their lives. Appropriate pretravel advice and screening, safe practices while abroad, and well-informed post-travel care can help to ensure that travelers return home with fond memories and an appetite for further international travel.

Paul S. Pottinger, MD, DTM&H, FIDSA
Division of Allergy and Infectious Diseases
Department of Medicine
University of Washington
Seattle, WA 98915, USA

Christopher A. Sanford, MD, MPH, DTM&H
Family Medicine, Global Health
University of Washington
Box 358732
Seattle, WA 98125, USA

E-mail addresses:
abx@u.washington.edu (P.S. Pottinger)
casanfo@uw.edu (C.A. Sanford)

The Ethics of Medical Volunteerism

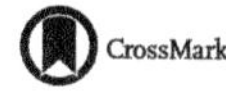

Geren S. Stone, MD, DTM&H*, Kristian R. Olson, MD, MPH, DTM&H

KEYWORDS

• Medical volunteerism • Medical mission • Ethics

KEY POINTS

- Thousands of health care providers volunteer annually for short-term medical service trips.
- These trips have the potential to both benefit and harm those involved.
- The context, resource and time limitations, and the language and cultural barriers present ethical challenges to volunteers.
- Based on published guidelines and program descriptions, we propose some guiding principles that can inform and equip those engaging in medical volunteerism including mission, partnership, preparation, reflection, support, sustainability, and evaluation.

BACKGROUND

In April 2014, the NY Times Opinion Pages hosted a debate titled "Can 'Voluntourism' make a difference?."[1] In response to the growing trend of travelers from high-income countries opting to volunteer in low resource settings, the investigators in this series of opinion pieces set forth their answers to the question based on their experience and expertise on the ethics and impact of short-term volunteers. Similarly, National Public Radio labeled "voluntourism" as "one of the fastest growing trends in travel today" with "more than 1.6 million volunteer tourists…spending about $2 billion each year" and asked the question "who's it helping most."[2] The NY Times and National Public Radio pieces portrayed growing tensions with this type of short-term service and detailed a mixture of opinions and perspectives on the benefits both for those serving and those being served.

Medical providers have a long history of volunteerism and service to those most in need. Short-term medical service trips (MSTs) have continued to grow in the recent

Disclosure: The authors have nothing to disclose.
Department of Medicine, MGH Center for Global Health, Massachusetts General Hospital, 55 Fruit Street, Boston, MA 02114, USA
* Corresponding author. Massachusetts General Hospital, MGH Global Health, Suite 722, 125 Nashua Street, Boston, MA 02114.
E-mail address: gstone@partners.org

Med Clin N Am 100 (2016) 237–246
http://dx.doi.org/10.1016/j.mcna.2015.09.001 medical.theclinics.com
0025-7125/16/$ – see front matter

past. Although no central monitoring body exists, researchers have found more than 500 organizations offering MSTs with a "very conservative estimate" of annual expenditures at $250 million.[3] These service trips last anywhere from days to months and are offered both by faith-based and non-faith-based organizations. They may be in response to disasters such as the recent earthquake in Nepal or the Ebola epidemic in West Africa, or focused on nonemergent health care in chronically underresourced areas. MSTs are especially common among students. In 2014, the Association of American Medical Colleges reported that 36% of matriculating medical students had participated in an international volunteer experience before medical school, and 29% of graduating medical students had participated in a global health rotation or volunteer experience during medical school.[4,5] These types of experiences are growing among all health professions and at all levels of training.

Although motivations for participating in MSTs vary by the individual, the underlying foundation is often a response to the health disparities and inequitable access to resources that exist globally. For instance, sub-Saharan Africa is estimated to have 24% of the global disease burden but only 2% of the global physician supply.[6] MSTs offer a means of response and opportunity to "do something." Therefore, investigators have written, "it is difficult to imagine a pursuit more closely aligned with the professional values and visceral instincts of most physicians."[7] Research has also described the benefits of such experiences for trainees, including a broadened medical knowledge, improved physical examination and procedural skills, enhanced sensitivity to cost issues, and a greater appreciation for cross-cultural communication.[8–20] Participants have demonstrated an increased likelihood to enter general primary care, obtain public health degrees, and engage in community service.[8,9,15]

Yet, in the midst of this growth of MSTs, there has been an increasing realization of the risks and challenges these experiences present. For participants, the risks can be to be their own personal health. In 1 study, 4% of participants in a medical program in Kenya experienced tuberculin skin test conversion after the experience.[21] Cultural differences may make communication and understanding difficult with respect to expectations, values, and decision making. Resources including equipment, personnel, and infrastructure are likely be limited compared with participants' usual work environment, requiring them to practice in new and unfamiliar ways, perhaps beyond the scope of their training and expertise, with pathologic conditions they may be unaccustomed to treating. For the host communities, these MSTs may pose safety risks to patients, compete with local services, and use limited local resources such as personnel and infrastructure based on external priorities and with little accountability. In the end, these short-term MSTs, although well intentioned, may actually cause harm leaving participants disenchanted and communities in a worse position than before.

Within this context, there has been an increasing call for dialogue about ethics and impact of short-term MSTs.[22–47] This article seeks to provide insight into the ethical challenges and offer some general principles from the literature to guide individuals and organizations involved in medical volunteerism.

ETHICAL CHALLENGES IN MEDICAL VOLUNTEER WORK

Context

There are many contextual features about medical volunteer work that can provide ethical challenges to volunteers. By the very nature of the work, volunteers travel to areas that lack resources including equipment, personnel, and infrastructure. This may be a short-term gap in the setting of a natural disaster or may be a longstanding shortage based on sociopolitical factors. Short-term volunteers may question the impact of MSTs that are only able to address the "symptoms of broader inequalities in health that require more radical solutions at the national and international level."[26] They may feel discouraged if they perceive themselves to only offer a 'band-aid,' while the deeper problems continue to exist.

The communities served by these MSTs are inherently vulnerable populations.[37] Whether victims of social, economic, or environmental factors, these communities have limited access to health care. Often impoverished, these populations are at risk of exploitation by MSTs, raising ethical concerns about informed consent, beneficence, coercion, autonomy, and justice. Exploitation may take place in various forms and to varying degrees, from the use of unauthorized patient photos for fund-raising and publicity to the extreme of practicing new procedural techniques during MSTs.[39,40] Volunteers in such settings may feel pressure and justification to work beyond the scope of their training and expertise based on the limited resources and the lack of other options for health care available to patients. In addition, patients may have limited understanding of the procedures and treatments including the risks of such plans as well as the qualifications of the health care provider offering the services.

In these settings, medical volunteers may encounter medical conditions that differ from those of their home context. Even when patients have familiar diseases, they often present at more advanced stages and may be complicated by conditions, such as severe malnutrition, for which medical volunteers may have limited experience.[22,32] Furthermore, the treatment options available to the volunteer may include medications or tools unfamiliar to them.

Limited Time and Resources

MSTs are limited in their duration. Testing and interventions often must be accomplished on a shortened timeline with limited availability for follow-up of outcomes including complications. The resources and equipment are often limited, leading health care providers to make diagnostic and treatment decisions very differently than they do in their usual practice. The overwhelming number of individuals in need may further complicate triage decisions, and the selection of patients to be seen and treated may become problematic. The process of triage may not be viewed by local stakeholders as transparent, equitable, or based on who is most in need of available services. The outcomes of MSTs reported to sponsors and the public are often measured in total numbers of patients seen and treated. This favors a "quantity over quality" approach limiting time with individuals.[32] With respect to MSTs providing surgical procedures, the emphasis on volume can overwhelm the health care system's ability to meet ongoing service needs.[22,23,32] Without intimate community knowledge or effective health record systems, follow-up care can be greatly compromised.

In addition, although often filling a short-term need, donations and other supplies brought in with MSTs may actually lead to delays in local leadership solving long-term supply problems. In fact, in response to the complexities of donating health care equipment, the World Health Organization has published guidelines as such donations can "even constitute an added burden to the recipient health care system" without proper planning and collaboration.[48]

Cultural and Language Barriers

All the above issues are compounded by cultural and language barriers. These barriers exist in daily domestic practice, but overseas they are often magnified, complicating communication and understanding of values, perceptions, and decision making. This can manifest as insufficient understanding of disease, including its causes and appropriate treatments.[32] Even when sharing a cultural background with a patient, it can be difficult to explain the risks and benefits of certain treatments and to reach a collaborative plan. Yet, communication and understanding are vital to providing patient-centered care, ensuring the patient's engagement in the treatment plan, and promoting the best health outcomes. Differences in culture and language can also complicate relationships between health care providers from different settings. Short-term volunteers may not understand how their decisions and recommendations conflict with the values and plans of local providers. This may lead to tension between host and visitor, and adversely impact the care of patients.

LESSONS FROM INTERNATIONAL RESEARCH

Parallels have been drawn between short-term medical volunteerism and international clinical research including the ethical considerations of each. International research ethics have become established over the last 2 decades. In 1997, a debate on the ethical standards of international research came to the forefront after a placebo-controlled clinical trial that was conducted in developing countries focused on the prevention of mother-to-child HIV transmission. In this case, controversy focused on the use of the placebo-controlled research design despite the existence of a proven efficacious standard of care.[49,50] Subsequently, in 1999, the Nuffield Council on Bioethics published their guidelines *The Ethics of Clinical Research in Developing Countries*.[51] The Nuffield Council and the Council for International Organizations of Medical Sciences ultimately agreed that patients involved in research should have the same standard of care provided as would be carried out in the research sponsor's country.[51,52]

In recent years, there have been calls for the application of similar guidelines to medical volunteer experiences.[26,30,34,53] Investigators have decried the lack of ethical frameworks and oversight for MSTs despite their significant operational similarities to international clinical research. They have even suggested the creation of a formalized ethical review process for MSTs involving the local community and similar to institutional review boards.[34]

PRINCIPLES FOR MEDICAL VOLUNTEERISM

Meanwhile, the literature on MSTs has been growing with respect to best practices and guidelines. Suchdev and colleagues,[54] based on their experience developing the Children's Health International Medical Project of Seattle, proposed the guiding principles of mission, collaboration, education, service, teamwork, sustainability, and evaluation. The Working Group on Ethics Guidelines for Training Experiences in Global Health's guidelines, published in 2010, further expanded these principles and best practices for institutions, students, and sponsors involved in such experiences during medical training.[30] Other programs and institutions have also published their curricula, guidelines, and organizational principles focused on the ethics of short-term MSTs.[35,43,55–57] In the realm of humanitarian assistance, the Sphere Project has developed the Core Humanitarian Standard (CHS).[58,59] CHS outlines a set of 9 commitments for both individuals and organizations to improve the quality and effectiveness of their interventions.[59] Together these guidelines and principles can be generally organized as mission, partnership, preparation, reflection, support, sustainability, and evaluation.

Mission

For an institution or an individual, a mission involves the purpose and motivation for service. This may be a formal mission statement that communicates a program's aims and values. For an individual, it may be less formal but is certainly no less valuable to consider, especially as each health care worker wants to work with an organization that reflects his or her own personal ethos and values. In general, the mission will encompass addressing global health disparities through service.

For an individual, however, the motivation to serve may also include a focus on personal growth and awareness. That is not to say, as some have written, that medical volunteerism should be seen as an alternative for tourism in order to see exotic places.[60] Personal growth does (and indeed should) accompany service in such environments. It is the relationships, experiences, and reflections that often leave participants stating, "I gained much more than I gave." Although this statement may sound self-centered and self-serving, it should be judged only in context with the benefits the communities received. During these experiences, the focus and priority should be given to the patients, but the health care providers and the communities can and should both benefit.

Partnership

As one author commented, even passionate, smart, and informed students may "make snap decisions about the best harmonization of complex [ethical and situational] concerns [in global health] without consulting the most important source of information: the people they serve."[55] Local collaboration and partnership are critical to MSTs. True collaborative partnerships begin with planning of the service, and carries on throughout the experience and beyond. It seeks to empower the local community, valuing their perspective and listening to their needs. As another author writes, part of the value in MSTs is the "expression of mutual caring or solidarity."[26] This type of partnership occurs through intentionally planning services that augment and support local priorities and values, rather than undermining or competing with them.

Whereas MSTs are often very brief, a long-term relationship is an important component of effective and sustainable delivery of quality patient care.[42] A long-term relationship may take different forms depending on each situation. Models may include MSTs with teams returning to the same location multiple times over the course of years or serving through an organization with a long-term staff on-site all year.

Preparation

Appropriate preparation for MSTs includes addressing individual health concerns and basic logistics, including volunteer safety, vaccinations, travel, and malpractice insurance. However, it also requires a basic understanding of local culture, health systems, epidemiology, and sociopolitical considerations.[30,42] It should focus on the practicalities of service in resource-limited settings and on principles of health equity, universality, and the socioeconomic determinants of health.[36,43] Preparation equips volunteers with a framework of expectations and tools to process the experiences and challenges. It may include informal discussion, formal didactic curricula, case studies, or simulation.[46,57,61]

Reflection

There is a growing emphasis on the need for personal reflection in order to process the experiences of MSTs, to maintain humility and openness, and to continue to provide the highest level of care.[38,57,61] Space and time for reflection allows room for personal growth as one becomes more aware of one's emotions, assumptions, biases, and values. The Ethics of International Engagement and Service Learning Project promotes a model of "reflective praxis" bringing together action and reflection.[61] For them, reflection "means critically examining one's own views, assumptions, convictions, and actions," and this practice "encourages thoughtful, careful, and evolving engagement."[61] Critical reflection promotes transformation, meaning, and connection in MSTs.

Support

Dialogue, mentorship, and social support are also vital components of short-term MSTs. Among humanitarian workers, burnout, depression, and substance abuse are common, with between 10% and 20% having reported depression, anxiety, or emotional exhaustion.[62] However, in 1 study, increased social support was associated with lower risk of depression or distress as well as greater life satisfaction.[62] Social support allows for a "continuous and open discussion" around challenges, stresses, and the benefits of service while also including clear communication protocols, supervision, and space for debriefing.[42] Mentorship and on-site coaching have been described as indispensable for MSTs.[55] Nevertheless, these components are frequently missing.[63]

Sustainability

Volunteers, institutions, and sponsors of MSTs should consider how their work is building beyond the short-term experience.[30] This may involve training local providers, building local infrastructure, and maintaining long-term relationships.[35,54] It must be built on local collaboration and an empowering partnership while being realistic about the limited time and funds characteristic of MSTs.[56,61]

Evaluation

Lastly, there are increasing calls for improvement in measurement and reporting the outcomes of MSTs. Although the field continues to grow, reports of the services are often anecdotal, narrative, or focused solely on the quantity of services offered.[41,45] Despite the thousands of trips and millions of dollars spent each year, 1 systematic review found only 6% of the published studies on MSTs over the last 20 years included even low-level evidence and data collection.[45] Organizations and institutions have a responsibility to those whom they send on MSTs, and the populations they serve, to ensure quality monitoring and evaluation. Sponsors and participants should require routine and ongoing measurements from organizations demonstrating the effectiveness of their MSTs.[30]

SUMMARY

> *Those who write and talk about the dream of global health equity can make people think, but can not make them care. It is only through direct involvement with the poor in the developing world (or here at home) that medical students and others in the medical profession at large will find reasons to care and, ultimately, find ways to change the health of the world's most vulnerable.*
>
> —*Edward O'Neil*[25]

Gustavo Gutiérrez, the father of liberation theology, once advised people to forget the "head trip" of studying the problems of the poor and take a "foot trip" to work among them.[25] Medical volunteering offers an opportunity for health care providers to take such a "foot trip." The experiences challenge, encourage, and change participants. They promote a sense of a "common humanity" and that "their suffering is our suffering."[26] Yet, there is a growing realization that, despite good intentions, these MSTs may fall short of their goals to address the inequities present and may even harm the very communities they are meant to serve. As health care professionals, we bear the social responsibility of our actions to serve the welfare of our patients and first and foremost to "do no harm."[64] The contexts, resource and time limitations, and the language and cultural barriers may present various ethical challenges to volunteers, and therefore there have been increasing calls for guidelines, transparency, and open review of MSTs and their outcomes. Parallels have been drawn to international research in developing countries for which guidelines and best practices have been formally developed and implemented over the last 2 decades. While the dialogue continues, principles of mission, partnership, preparation, reflection, support, sustainability, and evaluation can inform and equip those engaging in medical volunteerism. With thoughtfulness and humility, we can and should serve those in need, focused and reliant on collaboration, introspection, and ongoing dialogue to help us navigate this space filled with incredible complexity, challenge, and reward: both for those who serve and those who are served.

REFERENCES

1. NY Times, Can 'voluntourism' make a difference?, in the opinion pages: room for debate. 2014. Available online at: http://www.nytimes.com/roomfordebate/2014/04/29/can-voluntourism-make-a-difference.
2. Kahn C. As 'voluntourism' explodes in popularity, who's it helping most? In goats and soda: stories of life in a changing world. Washington, DC: National Public Radio; 2014.
3. Maki J, Qualls M, White B, et al. Health impact assessment and short-term medical missions: a methods study to evaluate quality of care. BMC Health Serv Res 2008;8:121.
4. Association of American Medical Colleges (AAMC). Matriculating student questionnaire: 2014 all schools summary report. Washington, DC: Association of American Medical Colleges; 2014.
5. Association of American Medical Colleges (AAMC). Medical school graduation questionnaire: 2014 all schools summary report. Washington, DC: Association of American Medical Colleges; 2014.
6. Scheffler RM, Liu JX, Kinfu Y, et al. Forecasting the global shortage of physicians: an economic- and needs-based approach. Bull World Health Organ 2008;86(7):516–523B.
7. Shaywitz DA, Ausiello DA. Global health: a chance for Western physicians to give-and receive. Am J Med 2002;113(4):354–7.
8. Miller WC, Corey GR, Lallinger GJ, et al. International health and internal medicine residency training: the Duke University experience. Am J Med 1995;99(3):291–7.
9. Gupta AR, Wells CK, Horwitz RI, et al. The international health program: the fifteen-year experience with Yale University's Internal Medicine Residency Program. Am J Trop Med Hyg 1999;61(6):1019–23.
10. Haq C, Rothenberg D, Gjerde C, et al. New world views: preparing physicians in training for global health work. Fam Med 2000;32(8):566–72.
11. Haskell A, Rovinsky D, Brown HK, et al. The University of California at San Francisco international orthopaedic elective. Clin Orthop Relat Res 2002;(396):12–8.

12. Thompson MJ, Huntington MK, Hunt DD, et al. Educational effects of international health electives on U.S. and Canadian medical students and residents: a literature review. Acad Med 2003;78(3):342–7.
13. Godkin M, Savageau J. The effect of medical students' international experiences on attitudes toward serving underserved multicultural populations. Fam Med 2003;35(4):273–8.
14. Mutchnick IS, Moyer CA, Stern DT. Expanding the boundaries of medical education: evidence for cross-cultural exchanges. Acad Med 2003;78(10 Suppl): S1–5.
15. Ramsey AH, Haq C, Gjerde CL, et al. Career influence of an international health experience during medical school. Fam Med 2004;36(6):412–6.
16. Federico SG, Zachar PA, Oravec CM, et al. A successful international child health elective: the University of Colorado Department of Pediatrics' experience. Arch Pediatr Adolesc Med 2006;160(2):191–6.
17. Disston AR, Martinez-Diaz GJ, Raju S, et al. The international orthopaedic health elective at the University of California at San Francisco: the eight-year experience. J Bone Joint Surg Am 2009;91(12):2999–3004.
18. Sawatsky AP, Rosenman DJ, Merry SP, et al. Eight years of the Mayo International Health Program: what an international elective adds to resident education. Mayo Clin Proc 2010;85(8):734–41.
19. Petrosoniak A, McCarthy A, Varpio L. International health electives: thematic results of student and professional interviews. Med Educ 2010;44(7):683–9.
20. Campbell A, Sherman R, Magee WP. The role of humanitarian missions in modern surgical training. Plast Reconstr Surg 2010;126(1):295–302.
21. Gardner A, Cohen T, Carter EJ. Tuberculosis among participants in an academic global health medical exchange program. J Gen Intern Med 2011;26(8):841–5.
22. Dupuis CC. Humanitarian missions in the third world: a polite dissent. Plast Reconstr Surg 2004;113(1):433–5.
23. Wolfberg AJ. Volunteering overseas–lessons from surgical brigades. N Engl J Med 2006;354(5):443–5.
24. White MT, Cauley KL. A caution against medical student tourism. Virtual Mentor 2006;8(12):851–4.
25. O'Neil E Jr. The "ethical imperative" of global health service. Virtual Mentor 2006; 8(12):846–50.
26. DeCamp M. Scrutinizing global short-term medical outreach. Hastings Cent Rep 2007;37(6):21–3.
27. Anderson FW, Wansom T. Beyond medical tourism: authentic engagement in global health. Virtual Mentor 2009;11(7):506–10.
28. Green T, Green H, Scandlyn J, et al. Perceptions of short-term medical volunteer work: a qualitative study in Guatemala. Global Health 2009;5:4.
29. Chapin E, Doocy S. International short-term medical service trips: guidelines from the literature and perspectives from the field. World Health Popul 2010;12(2): 43–53.
30. Crump JA, Sugarman J, Working Group T. on Ethics Guidelines for Global Health, Ethics and best practice guidelines for training experiences in global health. Am J Trop Med Hyg 2010;83(6):1178–82.
31. Jesus JE. Ethical challenges and considerations of short-term international medical initiatives: an excursion to Ghana as a case study. Ann Emerg Med 2010; 55(1):17–22.
32. Wall A. The context of ethical problems in medical volunteer work. HEC Forum 2011;23(2):79–90.

33. Langowski MK, Iltis AS. Global health needs and the short-term medical volunteer: ethical considerations. HEC Forum 2011;23(2):71–8.
34. DeCamp M. Ethical review of global short-term medical volunteerism. HEC Forum 2011;23(2):91–103.
35. Ott BB, Olson RM. Ethical issues of medical missions: the clinicians' view. HEC Forum 2011;23(2):105–13.
36. Snyder J, Dharamsi S, Crooks VA. Fly-By medical care: conceptualizing the global and local social responsibilities of medical tourists and physician voluntourists. Global Health 2011;7:6.
37. Wall LL. Ethical concerns regarding operations by volunteer surgeons on vulnerable patient groups: the case of women with obstetric fistulas. HEC Forum 2011; 23(2):115–27.
38. Abedini NC, Gruppen LD, Kolars JC, et al. Understanding the effects of short-term international service-learning trips on medical students. Acad Med 2012; 87(6):820–8.
39. Holt GR. Ethical conduct of humanitarian medical missions: I. informed consent. Arch Facial Plast Surg 2012;14(3):215–7.
40. Holt GR. Ethical conduct of humanitarian medical missions: II. use of photographic images. Arch Facial Plast Surg 2012;14(4):295–6.
41. Martiniuk AL, Manouchehrian M, Negin JA, et al. Brain gains: a literature review of medical missions to low and middle-income countries. BMC Health Serv Res 2012;12:134.
42. Asgary R, Junck E. New trends of short-term humanitarian medical volunteerism: professional and ethical considerations. J Med Ethics 2013;39(10): 625–31.
43. Saffran L. Dancing through cape coast: ethical and practical considerations for health-related service-learning programs. Acad Med 2013;88(9):1212–4.
44. Seymour B, Benzian H, Kalenderian E. Voluntourism and global health: preparing dental students for responsible engagement in international programs. J Dent Educ 2013;77(10):1252–7.
45. Sykes KJ. Short-term medical service trips: a systematic review of the evidence. Am J Public Health 2014;104(7):e38–48.
46. Logar T, Le P, Harrison JD, et al. Teaching corner: "first do no harm": teaching global health ethics to medical trainees through experiential learning. J Bioeth Inq 2015;12(1):69–78.
47. Kittle N, McCarthy V. Teaching corner: raising the bar: ethical considerations of medical student preparation for short-term immersion experiences. J Bioeth Inq 2015;12(1):79–84.
48. World Health Organization. Guidelines for Health Care Equipment Donations. Geneva (Switzerland): World Health Organization; 2000.
49. Angell M. The ethics of clinical research in the third world. N Engl J Med 1997; 337(12):847–9.
50. Lurie P, Wolfe SM. Unethical trials of interventions to reduce perinatal transmission of the human immunodeficiency virus in developing countries. N Engl J Med 1997;337(12):853–6.
51. Nuffield Council on Bioethics. The ethics of clinical research in developing countries. London: Nuffield Council on Bioethics; 1999.
52. Council for International Organizations of Medical Sciences. International ethical guidelines for biomedical research involving human subjects. Geneva (Switzerland): Council for International Organizations of Medical Sciences (CIOMS); 2002.

53. Shah S, Wu T. The medical student global health experience: professionalism and ethical implications. J Med Ethics 2008;34(5):375–8.
54. Suchdev P, Ahrens K, Click E, et al. A model for sustainable short-term international medical trips. Ambul Pediatr 2007;7(4):317–20.
55. Lahey T. Perspective: a proposed medical school curriculum to help students recognize and resolve ethical issues of global health outreach work. Acad Med 2012;87(2):210–5.
56. Heck JE, Bazemore A, Diller P. The shoulder to shoulder model-channeling medical volunteerism toward sustainable health change. Fam Med 2007;39(9): 644–50.
57. Sheather J, Shah T. Ethical dilemmas in medical humanitarian practice: cases for reflection from Medecins Sans Frontieres. J Med Ethics 2011;37(3):162–5.
58. The Sphere Project. The Sphere Project: humanitarian charter and minimum standards in humanitarian response. 3rd edition. Hampshire (United Kingdom): Hobbs the Printers; 2011.
59. The Sphere Project, The core humanitarian standards and the sphere core standards- analysis and comparison. Version 2 edition. Geneva (Switzerland): The Sphere Project; 2015.
60. Godfrey J, Wearing S, Schulenkorf N. Medical volunteer tourism as an alternative to backpacking in Peru. Tourism Planning and Development 2015;12(1):111–22.
61. The Ethics of International Engagement and Service Learning Project. Global praxis: exploring the ethics of engagement abroad. Vancouver (BC): The Ethics of International Engagement and Service-Learning Project; 2011.
62. Lopes Cardozo B, Gotway Crawford C, Eriksson C, et al. Psychological distress, depression, anxiety, and burnout among international humanitarian aid workers: a longitudinal study. PLoS One 2012;7(9):e44948.
63. Crump JA, Sugarman J. Guidelines for global health training. Health Aff 2011; 30(6):1215.
64. Smith CM. Origin and uses of primum non nocere–above all, do no harm! J Clin Pharmacol 2005;45(4):371–7.

Immunizations

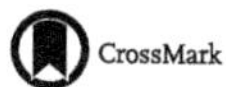

Christopher A. Sanford, MD, MPH, DTM&H[a,*],
Elaine C. Jong, MD, FIDSA, FASTMH[b]

KEYWORDS

- Immunizations • Vaccines • Pre-travel • Consultation • Preventative
- Travel medicine • Adventure medicine • Vaccinology

KEY POINTS

- The pretravel provider must address vaccine-preventable illnesses with every traveler and make vaccine recommendations based on travelers' past vaccination history, medical history, and anticipated itinerary and activities.
- As a general rule, domestic vaccine-preventable illnesses, including influenza and hepatitis A, are more common in international travelers than are exotic or low-income-nation-associated vaccine-preventative illnesses, such as typhoid fever or Japanese encephalitis; hence, pretravel providers should first ensure that travelers are current on domestic or routine immunizations.
- Additional immunizations may be indicated depending on a traveler's anticipated itinerary, activities, mode of travel, and length of stay.

Advising the traveler about vaccine-preventable diseases is a cornerstone of the pretravel consultation. In addition to ensuring that travelers are current regarding routine, or domestic vaccinations, pretravel providers may advise additional vaccinations depending on itinerary, mode of travel, anticipated activities, and duration of stay.

The approach to a patient regarding vaccines for travel is guided by understanding a few basic principles of immunization. Active immunization occurs when a person's immune system responds to specific antigens by producing antibodies: protection elicited by active immunization may last months or years, or be lifelong, depending on the antigen. Active immunity may be acquired either by surviving a natural infection or by receiving vaccination with disease-specific antigens.

Vaccine antigens consisting of live attenuated microorganisms (viruses or bacteria) generally produce the most robust immune responses compared with inactivated vaccines containing killed microorganisms or purified antigen derivatives. However, severe adverse vaccine-associated reactions are more likely with live vaccines than with inactivated ones. Live vaccines are biologically fragile and must be stored and

[a] Family Medicine, Global Health, University of Washington, Box 358732, Seattle, WA 98125, USA; [b] Division of Allergy & Infectious Diseases, Department of Medicine, University of Washington, 1100 4th Avenue S Edmonds, Seattle, WA 98020, USA
* Corresponding author.
E-mail address: casanfo@uw.edu

Med Clin N Am 100 (2016) 247–259
http://dx.doi.org/10.1016/j.mcna.2015.08.018 medical.theclinics.com

handled carefully in order to preserve efficacy, a challenge to the distribution of such vaccines in tropical climates (eg, measles-mumps-rubella vaccine). Vaccines using protein antigens or polysaccharide antigens coupled to protein carriers elicit a more durable response than polysaccharide antigens alone. Although inactivated and purified antigen derivative vaccines generally tend to have a lower adverse side effects profile in recipients compared with live vaccines, multiple doses are usually necessary to attain protective levels of antibody (eg, inactivated polio vaccine).

Passive immunization refers to the process by which a person receives immune protection by transfer of antibodies produced by another person or animal. This immunization provides temporary protection, as the passively transferred antibodies degenerate over time. An example of passive immunization is the protection of babies by antibodies passed from their mothers in the final 1 to 2 months of pregnancy. This protection lasts for up to 1 year. Another example of passive immunization is the administration of human immune globulin (IG), which was commonly given to travelers for protection against hepatitis A before the approval of the hepatitis A vaccine in 1995.

IG contains human antibodies derived by pooling the immunoglobulin G (IgG) antibody fraction from serum samples of thousands of donors. The antibodies contained in IG reflect the immune status of the donor pool and may differ from country to country. In the United States, IG usually contains antibodies against some of the vaccine-preventable diseases covered by the routine immunization programs (eg, tetanus, diphtheria, measles, mumps, rubella, polio, hepatitis A) as well as some of the prevalent communicable diseases, whereas IG prepared in Asia is more likely to contain antibodies against hepatitis B and hepatitis E.

Human hyperimmune globulin contains high titers of antibody against a specific disease pathogen and is used for postexposure prophylaxis in highly susceptible patients exposed to certain infectious diseases, such as hepatitis B (HBIG), rabies (RIG), and varicella (VZIG).[1]

ROUTINE VACCINES

Vaccine-preventable diseases addressed in public health programs for the routine immunization of infants, children, and adults, such as measles, hepatitis A, and influenza, are more commonly acquired by international travelers than are the more exotic travel diseases, such as typhoid fever and cholera. Thus, the starting point of counseling on travel immunizations during the pretravel encounter should be to verify that the traveler is up to date on the routine or domestic vaccinations and to identify if any booster doses are needed. The Advisory Committee on Immunization Practices (ACIP) at the Centers for Disease Control and Prevention (CDC) reviews vaccines licensed by the Food and Drug Administration (FDA) and makes annual recommendations for routine pediatric and adult immunization schedules in the United States, with interim updates as needed. The ACIP also reviews travel and special vaccines. The vaccine schedules, recommendations, and updates are available at http://www.cdc.gov.

Tetanus, Diphtheria, Pertussis

Cases of tetanus, pertussis, and diphtheria are more common in low-income nations because of suboptimal vaccine coverage. Children should receive the primary series of 5 doses of diphtheria, tetanus, and acellular pertussis (whooping cough) at 2, 4, 6, and 15 to 18 months of age and at 4 to 6 years of age. Tetanus and diphtheria (Td) should be given to adolescents and adults as a booster dose every 10 years. The tetanus toxoid, reduced diphtheria toxoid, and acellular pertussis vaccine (Tdap), which also includes protection against pertussis, should be given to adolescents at 11 to 18 years of age instead of Td. Adults 19 years of age and older should receive a single dose of Tdap instead of a booster dose of Td if they did not receive Tdap as an adolescent. Pregnant women should receive a dose of Tdap during each pregnancy, ideally between 27 and 36 weeks of gestation. Tdap can be administered without regard to when the most recent Td was administered.

Measles, Mumps, Rubella

Measles, mumps, and rubella (MMR) are all more common in low-income nations where childhood immunization programs are not fully implemented. In 2013, measles caused an estimated 146,000 deaths globally,[1] most of them in children younger than 5 years in Africa. Measles was eliminated in the United States in 2000. (Elimination is defined as the absence of continuous disease transmission for 12 months or more in a specific geographic area.) Since then, the number of cases per year in the United States has ranged from a low of 37 in 2004 to a high of 644 in 2014. Between January 1 and March 27, 2015, 178 cases were reported. Most people who contracted measles were unvaccinated[2]; some had recently returned from foreign travel. Children older than 12 months should receive 2 doses of the MMR vaccine, separated by at least 28 days. Infants 6 to 11 months of age traveling to regions of elevated risk for these 3 diseases may receive a single dose of MMR. However, this dose does not count; the infant still requires 2 additional doses, separated by at least 28 days, after 1 year of age. Two doses of the MMR vaccine separated by at least 28 days should be administered to nonimmune adults born in or after 1957. About 95% of vaccine recipients become immune after a single dose of vaccine administered after 1 year of age; this increases to more than 99% of those receiving 2 doses.

Rotavirus

Globally, rotavirus is a common cause of severe diarrhea in young children, causing 2 million hospitalizations and half a million deaths annually of children younger than 5 years. Vaccination for rotavirus is given to young infants orally: either 3 doses of the live, oral, pentavalent rotavirus vaccine (RV5) at 2, 4, and 6 months of age or 2 doses of live, oral rotavirus vaccine (RV1) at 2 and 4 months of age.

For several reasons, including concurrent enteric infections and malnutrition, oral vaccines are less efficacious in low-income nations. Rotavirus vaccine was found to be 98% protective in Finnish children but only 58% protective in Nicaraguan children and 46% protective in Bangladeshi children.[3]

Polio

The primary immunization schedule for polio is a 4-dose series, given at 2, 4, and 6 to 18 months of age plus a booster dose at 4 to 6 years of age. In the United States, inactivated poliovirus vaccine (IPV) administered by injection is the only vaccine formulation used; oral live attenuated polio vaccine is used in some countries outside the United States.

Polio remains endemic in 2 nations: Afghanistan and Pakistan; a small number of cases are reported in additional countries. Adults who received the complete pediatric series should receive a single additional dose of IPV before travel to destinations where polio may be in circulation: Afghanistan, Cameroon, Equatorial Guinea, Ethiopia, Iraq, Israel, the West Bank and Gaza, Nigeria, Pakistan, Somalia, and Syria. A single additional dose is also advised for those with a high risk of exposure to polio (eg, someone working in a health care setting or in a refugee camp) in Benin, Central African Republic, Chad, China (Xinjiang province only), Djibouti, Egypt, Eritrea, Gabon, Iran, Jordan, Kenya, Lebanon, Niger, Republic of Congo, South Sudan, Sudan, Turkey, and Yemen.[4] Repeat boosters of polio vaccine after the single booster dose received as an adult are not advised. The nations for which polio vaccine is advised are prone to change; the CDC Web site (http://www.cdc.gov) or the World Health Organization (WHO) Web site (http://www.who.int) should be consulted for the current list.[5]

Hepatitis A

Hepatitis A, transmitted by consuming fecally contaminated food or beverages, is one of the most common vaccine-preventable illnesses among international travelers to low-income nations. Although 70% of cases in children younger than 6 years are asymptomatic, older children and adults may experience debilitating symptoms lasting for 2 to 8 weeks or longer. The case-fatality rate in those older than 50 years is 2.7%.[6]

The inactivated hepatitis A vaccine series consists of 2 doses, separated by at least 6 months, administered by injection. There is no need for subsequent boosters. The minimum age to receive hepatitis A vaccine is 1 year old.

Hepatitis B

Hepatitis B is transmitted by blood, blood products, and body fluids, including semen. Travelers may be exposed by unprotected sex, undergoing medical procedures whereby blood products may not be screened for hepatitis B or instruments are not properly sterilized, or by receiving tattoos or acupuncture with unsterilized equipment. The inactivated hepatitis B vaccine series consists of 3 doses (at 0, 1, and 6 months) administered by injection. An accelerated schedule of hepatitis B vaccine may be considered for travelers leaving on short notice who face potential exposure (eg, medical providers traveling to respond to a disaster); this consists of doses at days 0, 7, and 21 to 30, plus a fourth dose at 1 year. Also, the accelerated schedule for the hepatitis A and B combination vaccine might be considered for travelers who need protection against hepatitis A and B; this consists of doses on days 0, 7, and 21 to 30, plus a fourth dose at 1 year.

Haemophilus Influenzae Type b

Haemophilus influenzae type b (Hib) is a bacterium that causes meningitis, pneumonia, and other infections, usually in children younger than 5 years. Three monovalent Haemophilus influenzae type b (Hib) conjugate vaccines are licensed in the United States. Hib conjugate vaccines are also available in combination with other vaccines. Hib conjugate vaccine is administered as either 3 or 4 doses, depending on the vaccine brand, with doses at 2, 4, 6 (if needed, depending on vaccine brand), and 12 to 15 months (final/booster dose). The Hib conjugate vaccine is also available as a component of several combination vaccines. Usually, those older than 5 years do not require this vaccine. However, it is sometimes administered to older children and adults with chronic conditions associated with an increased risk of Hib disease, for example, splenectomized, sickle cell disease, and following leukemia chemotherapy or bone marrow transplant. Sometimes, Hib conjugate vaccine is also administered to human immunodeficiency virus (HIV)-positive individuals between 5 and 18 years of age.

Human Papillomavirus

Human papillomavirus (HPV) infections are the most common sexually transmitted infections in the United States. There are more than 40 HPV types, and immunization against HPV infection is a public health priority because some high-risk HPV types cause cervical cancer, anal cancer, oropharyngeal cancers, and rarer cancers (eg, vaginal, vulvar, penile). Low-risk HPV types do not cause cancer but can cause skin warts on or around the genitals, anus, mouth, or throat.

In 2014, a 9-valent HPV vaccine was approved for use in the United States by the FDA; in 2015, the ACIP recommended this vaccine as one of the 3 HPV vaccines that may be used for routine vaccination (in addition to the bivalent vaccine, and HPV quadrivalent recombinant vaccine).[7] Routine vaccination with the 3 dose-series is advised for both girls and boys starting at 11 or 12 years of age, but the HPV vaccine may be given at as young as 9 years of age. The 3 doses are administered at 0, 1 to 2, and 6 months by injection. The HPV vaccine may be given up to 26 years of age in women and up to 21 years of age in men. It is also advised for men who have sex with men, and immunocompromised men, up to 26 years of age. Ideally all 3 doses are administered before an individual's sexual debut.

Influenza

Influenza is the most common vaccine-preventable disease in international travelers.[8] Between 1976 and 2007, a range between a low of 3000 and a high of 49,000 people in the United States died each year of influenza. Approximately 90% of those who died were older than 65 years. In the Northern Hemisphere (eg, the United States), the annual influenza season starts as early as October and can last as late as April or May; in the temperate regions of the Southern Hemisphere (eg, Australia), the season is opposite, usually occurring during April to September. In the tropics, influenza occurs year-round.

Vaccination is indicated for almost everyone older than 6 months of age without contraindications. Vaccination with inactivated influenza vaccine given by injection or with live attenuated influenza vaccine given by intranasal spray are equally effective. Despite the universal recommendation that everyone older than 6 months receive immunization for influenza, coverage rates for many groups remains low. A study conducted at a New York University published in 2015 found that only 28% of students had coverage.[9]

Meningococcal Disease

The bacterium *Neisseria meningitidis*, or meningococcus, causes meningitis, sepsis, and other illnesses. The incidence of meningococcal meningitis is highest in the meningitis belt of sub-Saharan Africa, with epidemics occurring there during the dry season of December to -June. Risk is also elevated in those residing in crowded living situations, such as college dorms or military barracks.

Currently 3 vaccines for meningococcal disease are licensed in the United States. Two are quadrivalent (serogroups A, C, Y, W135) meningococcal capsular polysaccharide–protein conjugate vaccines; the third vaccine is a quadrivalent meningococcal capsular polysaccharide vaccine, which is licensed for those 2 to 55 years of age. A 2-dose primary series of Menactra is licensed for children aged 9 to 23 months; a 1-dose primary series of Menactra is licensed for those 2 to 55 years of age. Menevo is licensed for those aged 2 to 55 years. Routine vaccination at 11 to 12 years of age with the conjugate vaccine, with a booster dose at 16 years of age, is now advised. For those receiving their first dose at 13 to 15 years of age, a single booster dose is advised at 16 to 18 years of age. A booster dose is not advised for those who receive their first dose after 16 years of age unless they continue to have an elevated risk for meningococcal disease.

The Saudi Arabian government requires those entering the country for the purpose of umrah or pilgrimage (hajj) to demonstrate proof of vaccination with a tetravalent vaccine (A, C, Y, W135) for meningococcal meningitis no more than 3 years and no less than 10 days before entry.[10] Some travelers previously vaccinated for meningococcal meningitis who are living in or returning to Africa's meningitis belt require booster doses. Those 9 months through 6 years of age should receive a conjugate booster 3 years after their previous dose and a booster dose every 5 years thereafter if at an increased risk. Those previously vaccinated at 7 to 55 years of age who remain at an elevated risk should receive an additional dose of conjugate vaccine 5 years after the previous dose and at 5-year intervals thereafter. Those older than 55 years should be vaccinated or revaccinated with the polysaccharide vaccine if more than 5 years have elapsed since their most recent meningococcal vaccine.

Two vaccines against *Neisseria meningitidis* group B have been licensed in the United States recently for disease prevention during specific meningococcal B outbreak situations and for persons engaged in certain high-risk occupations (eg, laboratory workers). Bexsara is given as 2 doses 1 month apart administered by injection. TruMemba is given as a series of 3 doses on 0, 2, and 6 months, administered by injection. In 2015, the ACIP voted to follow the recommendation of ACIP's meningococcal working group, which stated that the serogroup B meningococcal vaccine series may be administered to adolescents and young adults 16 through 23 years of age, further specifying that 16 to 18 years is the preferred age for vaccination. However, at the time of writing, meningococcal B vaccine was not recommended for incorporation into the standard childhood immunization schedules or for routine administration to students going to live on college campuses in the United States. This vaccine might be an appropriate consideration for certain travelers, such as health care providers and aid workers going to work in outbreak areas.

Pneumococcal Disease

The *Streptococcus pneumoniae* bacteria causing pneumococcal disease are transmitted person to person via respiratory droplets and have a worldwide distribution but are more common in low-income nations. *S pneumonia* infections are a common cause of pneumonia, meningitis, and septicemia, which can lead to life-threatening illness. Vaccines against pneumococcal disease incorporate the bacterial serotypes that are particularly associated with serious invasive disease and are prepared from purified pneumococcal polysaccharides (PPS). Pneumococcal conjugate vaccines are prepared from PPS conjugated to a protein carrier and are now recommended for primary immunization because the conjugate vaccines have increased immunogenicity compared with the PPS vaccines.

Pneumococcal conjugate vaccine, PCV13 is advised for all children younger than 5 years of age, adults older than 65 years, and those 6 to 64 years of age with certain medical conditions. The 4-dose series is given to infants at 2, 4, 6, and 12 to 15 months of age.

Pneumococcal polysaccharide vaccine, PPSV23, is recommended for adults older than 65 years and for those older than 2 years who are at an elevated risk for pneumococcal disease (including those with sickle cell disease, HIV infection, or immunosuppression from other causes). It is also advised for adults 19 to 64 years of age who smoke tobacco or have asthma.

Previously only PPSV23 was advised for those older than 65 years; however, in 2014 the ACIP recommended that this group also receive PCV13. For those older than 65 years who have received neither PCV13 nor PPSV23, the dose of PCV13 should be followed by a dose of PPSV23 after an interval of 6 to 12 months. For those older than 65 years who have received at least one dose of PPSV23 but not PCV13, a dose of PCV13 should be given at least 1 year after the most recent dose of PPSV23.[11]

Varicella (Chickenpox)

In temperate climes, for example, the United States, varicella is most common in preschool and school-aged children. In tropical climates, infection tends to occur later in childhood and during adolescence, causing a higher susceptibility in adults relative to temperate regions. Children younger than 13 years should receive 2 doses of varicella vaccine, a live attenuated virus vaccine administered by injection: the first at 12 to 15 months of age and the second at 4 to 6 years of age. Those 13 years of age and older should receive 2 doses at least 28 days apart.

Those with a reliable history of having had varicella do not need to be immunized. If there is uncertainty regarding past infection, options are obtaining a varicella-zoster IgG antibody assay (and immunizing those who test negative) or immunizing despite the possibility of preexisting protection. (As a general rule, immunizing a person with a vaccine for a disease to which the person is already immune does not cause harm.)

Zoster (Shingles)

Approximately one person in 3 will develop zoster (shingles) during his or her lifetime. The etiologic agent of varicella and zoster is one and the same. Varicella is the primary infection caused by the etiologic agent, varicella-zoster virus (VZV). Once this infection resolves, the virus is not cleared from the body but remains dormant in the dorsal root ganglia. The virus may then reactivate later in life to cause zoster. Hence, both varicella and zoster cases can transmit the virus to a previously unexposed person causing varicella but not zoster; one only develops zoster from a previous varicella infection. Zoster manifests as a painful unilateral vesicular rash, often in a dermatomal distribution. Approximately 10% to 18% of those with an attack of zoster will develop long-term pain from the episode of VZV reactivation termed postherpetic neuralgia.[12]

Immunization against zoster, which consists of a single dose of zoster vaccine at 60 years of age or older, is advised for most adults. Contraindications to immunization with zoster include significant immunosuppression due to HIV/AIDS, prolonged use of high-dose steroids, or other causes. Prior zoster infections are not a contraindication to immunization.

TRAVEL VACCINES

Typhoid Fever

The etiologic agent of typhoid fever is *Salmonella enterica*, serovar Typhi, which is transmitted by consuming contaminated food and beverages (fecal-oral route of spread). Typhoid fever is common in low-income nations; globally it causes an estimated 21 million infections and 200,000 deaths each year. Of the approximately 6000 cases that occur in the United States each year, up to 75% are acquired while traveling internationally. Although longer duration of stay abroad and more rustic or rural travel is associated with an increased risk of typhoid fever, this illness has been contracted after even very brief stays in low-income nations. The most frequent region in which travelers acquire typhoid fever is South Asia (the Indian subcontinent).[13] Symptoms include high fever, headache, abdominal pain, weakness, dry cough, anorexia, diarrhea or constipation, and sometimes a rash, which can be difficult to discern in dark-skinned people.

There is both an oral live attenuated vaccine and an injectable inactivated vaccine available for typhoid fever. The oral vaccine, which is indicated for travelers older than 6 years, consists of 4 tablets, taken one tablet every other day until completed. The tablets require refrigeration. The injectable form consists of one dose, administered intramuscularly; it is approved for travelers older than 2 years. The duration of protection for the oral form is 5 years and 2 years for the injectable form. Although these vaccines offer protection to many, overall efficacy for each is only 50% to 80%. The term *enteric fever* refers to both typhoid and paratyphoid fever; vaccination for typhoid fever only offers protection from the former.

Japanese Encephalitis

Japanese encephalitis (JE) is a mosquito-borne viral illness endemic to Asia and the Western Pacific. The virus reservoir hosts include domestic pigs and wild aquatic birds; the *Culex* mosquito vectors breed in the ubiquitous irrigated farmlands. Although uncommonly reported in travelers, it is a serious illness: of those who are symptomatic, approximately one-third fully recover, one-third are left with permanent neurologic sequelae, and one-third die. From 1973 through 2011, there were 58 published reports of travel-associated JE among travelers from nonendemic countries. From the time of licensure of a JE vaccine in the United States in 1992 through 2011, only 7 JE cases among US travelers were reported to the CDC.[14]

A purified inactivated JE virus vaccine derived from vaccine virus strains grown in Vero cell tissue cultures was licensed in the United States in 2009. Immunization consists of 2 doses separated by at least 28 days; the minimum age to receive this vaccine is 2 months. An accelerated vaccine schedule giving 2 doses 1 week apart has been published and showed noninferiority of the accelerated schedule compared with the standard schedule; however, the accelerated JE vaccine schedule is not licensed at the time of writing.[15] Regarding boosters, for those older than 17 years of age, if the primary series of 2 doses was administered over a year previously, a booster dose may be given if ongoing exposure to JE is anticipated. Safety and efficacy of boosters in those younger than 17 years has not been determined. A study published in 2015 indicated that 6 years after the booster dose of the purified inactivated JE virus vaccine, 96% of vaccine recipients has protective levels of antibodies; the averaged duration of protection after the booster dose was projected to be 14 years.[16]

The risk of JE exposure is higher for long-stay (more than 1 month) travelers to endemic areas, especially those going to visit, live, or work in rural or farming communities in endemic areas, than for short-stay travelers whose trips are limited to the urban environs. However, all travelers to JE endemic areas regardless of the length of stay should be educated about the risks of exposure (infected mosquito bites), self-protection measures against mosquito bites, and the availability of a safe efficacious vaccine to prevent JE, because the borders between urban and agricultural areas are often blurred in the transmission zones. There is a seasonal variation in incidence, which varies by country; a list of transmission seasons by nation is listed, in both online and print versions, in the CDC *Yellow Book*.[17]

Rabies

Rabies is a viral illness transmitted by the bite, scratch, or lick of an infected mammal. Once symptoms develop, the fatality rate is very close to 100%. In low-income nations, most cases of rabies are caused by the bites of domesticated animals, specifically dogs. Thirty-six deaths from rabies were reported in the United States between 1980 and 2000; about one-third of these were contracted overseas.[18]

Two inactivated tissue-culture–derived rabies vaccines licensed in the United States. Primary immunization consists of a series of 3 doses of vaccine administered by injection on days 0, 7, and 21 to 28. The need for boosters depends on the traveler's risk group. For most travelers, no booster is advised. However, for those at elevated risk of rabies, including spelunkers, veterinarians and staff, and animal control and wildlife workers in rabies-epizootic areas, periodic serologic testing is advised, with booster administration should antibody levels decrease to less than a protective threshold.

The postexposure series, in those who have completed the preexposure series, consists of 2 doses of rabies vaccine at days 0 and 3. In those who have not had the preexposure series, the CDC ACIP recommends a postexposure series of 4 doses of rabies vaccine (on days 0, 3, 7, and 14) or 5 doses of vaccine (on days 0, 3, 7, 14, and 30) (WHO schedule). A single dose of RIG is also required by both the CDC and WHO postexposure protocols, but this may not be readily accessible in low-income nations. The benefit of the WHO schedule is that it serves as preexposure series for potential subsequent exposures, whereas the efficacy of the ACIP schedule for this function is unclear.

Yellow Fever

Yellow fever is a viral illness transmitted by mosquitoes. It is present in 2 large geographic areas, in tropical Africa and tropical South America. It is not present in Asia. Hallmarks of this illness are jaundice (hence its moniker) and fever. The case-fatality rate for those who progress to hepatorenal dysfunction is 20% to 50%.

A highly efficacious vaccine has existed since the 1920s. Although current international regulations require proof of vaccination within the previous 10 years at many international borders within endemic regions, it has been known for many years that a single immunization of yellow fever vaccine provides lifelong immunity. This knowledge is slowly being incorporated into international regulations.

In 2013, an article in the WHO's *Weekly Epidemiologic Record* stated that WHO's Strategic Advisory Group of Experts on Immunizations (SAGE), after reviewing evidence, concluded that a single dose of yellow fever vaccine confers life-long immunity. In coming years, individual nations' regulations regarding demonstrating proof of vaccination for yellow fever may change to reflect the conclusions of WHO's SAGE. However, policy changes usually lag many years behind research findings. For now, travelers should assume that a border official requesting proof of vaccination will require that it have been within the previous 10 years.[19]

Yellow fever vaccine is a live attenuated virus vaccine derived from chick embryo cultures. It administered as a single dose by injection, and immune protection begins 10 days after receipt of the vaccine. The vaccine is contraindicated in persons with a history of anaphylactic shock following exposure to eggs or egg products, and the usual minimum age for administration is 9 months. The elderly are at elevated risk of adverse effects of yellow fever vaccine, including the rare but life-threatening yellow fever vaccine-associated viscerotropic disease. For elderly travelers who may require proof of yellow fever vaccination to cross international borders, but have minimal or no exposure to the disease, medical providers should not administer the vaccine but instead complete the waiver section of the traveler's International Certificate of Vaccination or Prophylaxis (yellow card). Other travelers for whom completion of the waiver section is preferable to vaccination include pregnant women and those who are immunocompromised. The CDC maintains a complete online list of contraindications for each vaccine.[20]

Travelers should carry their immunization records with their passports, so that they can display proof of immunization for yellow fever to customs officials if requested to do so.

VACCINES THAT ARE NOT ROUTINELY ADMINISTERED IN THE UNITED STATES

Tick-borne Encephalitis

Tick-borne encephalitis (TBE) is a viral infection transmitted by ticks in much of Europe, the former Soviet Union, and Asia. In endemic areas, those with recreational or occupational exposure to rural or outdoor settings (hikers, hunters, campers, farmers) are at risk for infection. No TBE vaccines are available in the United States; but several vaccines are licensed and available in Canada, Europe, and elsewhere. The routine primary vaccine series requires at least 6 months; hence, most travelers to TBE-endemic areas find that avoiding tick bites is more practical than receiving the vaccine. An accelerated vaccine schedule for both of the vaccines available in Europe has resulted in seroconversion rates similar to those following the standard vaccine schedule. Travelers at an elevated risk (those camping in endemic areas or those living in TBE-endemic countries for extended periods) may choose to be vaccinated in Canada or Europe.

Tuberculosis

Bacillus Calmette–Guérin (BCG) is a live attenuated vaccine for tuberculosis (TB). It is given to newborns in many countries with a high prevalence of TB. It has been shown to reduce the risk of TB meningitis and miliary disease.

The CDC recommends that BCG vaccine be administered only to those who meet specific criteria, in consultation with an expert in TB. It should be considered in children who are purified protein derivative (PPD) negative (and cannot be given long-term treatment of infection) who are continually exposed to, or cannot be separated from, adults who either are untreated or ineffectively treated for TB disease or have TB that is resistant to isoniazid and rifampin. It should only be considered in health care workers who work in a setting in which a high percentage of patients are infected with strains of TB resistant to both isoniazid and rifampin, or who work in a setting with ongoing transmission of drug-resistant TB, or in a setting in which TB infection-control measures have been implemented but have not been successful.[21]

Cholera

No cholera vaccine is licensed in the United States. The CDC does not recommend cholera vaccine for US travelers. An oral inactivated cholera vaccine is available in Canada, Western Europe, and Asia. Travelers to high-risk destinations may consider vaccination for cholera.

Oral Polio Virus

Oral live attenuated polio vaccine is given in many nations. It has not been used in the United States since 2000.

Smallpox

Naturally occurring smallpox disease has been eradicated. The last reported case in the United States was in 1949; the last naturally occurring case occurred in Somalia in 1977. Although some individuals continue to receive this vaccine (smallpox virus researchers, certain military personnel), this vaccine is not advised for international travelers and is not commercially available.

ADDITIONAL CLINICAL CONSIDERATIONS

Live Vaccines

Live vaccines include measles, mumps, rubella, polio (oral); rotavirus; varicella-zoster; influenza (intranasal); typhoid fever (oral); yellow fever; BCG (for TB); and smallpox. Typhoid fever (oral) and BCG are attenuated bacterial vaccines; the others on this list are attenuated viral vaccines. Pregnant women and those with immunosuppression should not receive live vaccines. Regarding those on chronic oral steroid therapy, many clinicians draw a line at 20 mg/d of prednisone or its equivalent, such that those taking less than that may receive live immunizations and those taking that dosage or higher do not.

Vaccine Interactions

Live viral vaccines should be administered on the same day, or at least 4 weeks apart to avoid an immune phenomenon known as viral interference Antibody-containing products (IG and homologous human hyperimmune globulin products [VZIG, HBIG, RIG]) may interfere with the response to live vaccines, including MMR. After administering a live viral vaccine, at least 2 weeks should elapse before an antibody-containing product is administered. After administering an antibody-containing product, the duration before a live viral vaccine can be administered varies depending on the dose of antibody; but a separation of at least 3 months is usually advised.[22] Regarding live viral vaccines and placing a PPD skin test for tuberculosis testing: this should be done on the same day or, after giving a live viral vaccine, at least 4 to 6 weeks should elapse before placing a PPD.

Vaccine Hesitancy

Many travelers are reluctant to agree to receive advised immunizations because of, among other reasons, concern regarding adverse effects. This phenomenon, termed *vaccine hesitancy*, is the result of a confluence of social, cultural, political, and personal factors.[23] Many people overestimate the potential risk from vaccines and underestimate the risk from infectious diseases. Some harbor misinformation, such as the belief that immunization for measles elevates the risk of autism, despite multiple large well-controlled studies having found no relationship between measles vaccine, or other vaccines, and autism.[24]

Some are reluctant to receive many immunizations at the same time because of a concern that their immune system may be overwhelmed. Patients should be counseled that studies show that receiving multiple simultaneous vaccines does not decrease efficacy, does not increase the risk of adverse effects, and in no way overwhelms the immune system.

Medical providers should be frank with travelers regarding potential adverse effects of vaccination but should also point out that for each vaccine that is advised, the odds of benefit from protection from disease is markedly higher than the risk from the vaccine.

REFERENCES

1. WHO. Measles fact sheet. 2015. Available at: http://www.who.int/mediacentre/factsheets/fs286/en/. Accessed June 5, 2015.
2. CDC: frequently asked questions about measles in the U.S. Available at: http://www.cdc.gov/measles/about/faqs.html. Accessed June 3, 2015.
3. Kirkpatrick BD, Colgate ER, Mychaleckyj JC, et al. The "Performance of Rotavirus and Oral Polio Vaccines in Developing Countries" (PROVIDE) Study: description

of methods of an interventional study designed to explore complex biologic problems. Am J Trop Med Hyg 2015;92(4):744–51.

4. CDC clinical update: polio vaccine guidance for travelers and note on travel to Israel, the West Bank, and Gaza. Available at: http://wwwnc.cdc.gov/travel/news-announcements/polio-vaccine-guidance-israel. Accessed May 14, 2015.
5. Clinical update: polio vaccine guidance for travelers and note on travel to Israel, the West Bank, and Gaza. Available at: http://wwwnc.cdc.gov/travel/news-announcements/polio-vaccine-guidance-israel. Accessed May 15, 2015.
6. American Liver Foundation: hepatitis A policy. Available at: http://www.liverfoundation.org/about/advocacy/hepapolicy/. Accessed June 2, 2015.
7. Petrosky E, Bocchini JA Jr, Hariri S, et al. Use of 9-valent human papillomavirus (HPV) vaccine: updated HPV vaccination recommendations of the advisory committee on immunization practices. MMWR Morb Mortal Wkly Rep 2015;64(11):300–4. Available at: http://www.cdc.gov/mmwr/preview/mmwrhtml/mm6411a3.htm#Tab1. Accessed June 2, 2015.
8. Steffen R. Influenza in travelers: epidemiology, risk, prevention, and control issues. Curr Infect Dis Rep 2010;12(3):181–5.
9. Bednarczyk RA, Chu SL, Sickler H, et al. Low uptake of influenza vaccine among university students: evaluating predictors beyond cost and safety concerns. Vaccine 2015;33(14):1659–63.
10. Royal embassy of Saudi Arabia: consular and travel services: hajj and umrah health requirements. Available at: http://www.saudiembassy.net/services/Hajj_and_Umrah_Health_Requirements.aspx. Accessed June 2, 2015.
11. Crawford, Chris: ACIP recommends routine PCV13 immunization for adults 65 and older. Available at: http://www.aafp.org/news/health-of-the-public/20140827pcv13vote.html. Accessed June 15, 2015.
12. Weaver BA. Herpes zoster overview: natural history and incidence. J Am Osteopath Assoc 2009;109(6 Suppl 2):S2–6.
13. Connor BA, Schwartz E. Typhoid and paratyphoid fever in travellers. Lancet Infect Dis 2005;5(10):623–8.
14. Hills SL, Weber IB, Fischer M. Japanese encephalitis. CDC health information for international travelers (yellow book). Available at: http://wwwnc.cdc.gov/travel/yellowbook/2014/chapter-3-infectious-diseases-related-to-travel/japanese-encephalitis. Accessed June 2, 2015.
15. Jellinek T, Burchard GD, Dieckmann S, et al. Short-term immunogenicity and safety of an accelerated pre-exposure prophylaxis regimen with Japanese encephalitis vaccine in combination with a rabies vaccine: a phase III, multicenter, observer-blind study. J Travel Med 2015;22:225–31.
16. Paulke-Korinek M, Kollaritsch H, Kundi M, et al. Persistence of antibodies six years after booster vaccination with inactivated vaccine against Japanese encephalitis. Vaccine 2015;33(30):3600–4.
17. Infectious diseases related to travel: Japanese encephalitis. Available at: http://wwwnc.cdc.gov/travel/yellowbook/2014/chapter-3-infectious-diseases-related-to-travel/japanese-encephalitis. Accessed June 15, 2015.
18. Arguin PM, Krebs JW, Mandel E, et al. Survey of rabies preexposure and postexposure prophylaxis among missionary personnel stationed outside the United States. J Travel Med 2000;7(1):10–4.
19. Vaccines and vaccination against yellow fever. Wkly Epidemiol Rec 2013;88(27):269–84. Available at: http://www.who.int/wer/2013/wer8827.pdf?ua=1. Accessed June 3, 2015.

20. CDC. Available at: http://www.cdc.gov/vaccines/vpd-vac/should-not-vacc.htm#shingles. Accessed May 15, 2015.
21. CDC: tuberculosis fact sheet: BCG vaccine. Available at: http://www.cdc.gov/tb/publications/factsheets/prevention/bcg.htm. Accessed June 1, 2015.
22. CDC: epidemiology and prevention of vaccine-preventable diseases (the pink book): general recommendations on immunizations. Available at: http://www.cdc.gov/vaccines/pubs/pinkbook/downloads/genrec.pdf. Accessed June 4, 2015.
23. Kestenbaum LA, Feemster KA. Identifying and addressing vaccine hesitancy. Pediatr Ann 2015;44(4):e71–5.
24. Jain A, Marshall J, Buikema A, et al. Autism occurrence by MMR vaccine status among us children with older siblings with and without autism. JAMA 2015;313(15):1534–40.

Travel Medical Kit

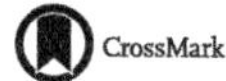

Anne C. Terry, RN, MSN, ARNP, N. Jean Haulman, MD, MPH*

KEYWORDS

- Travel medical kit • Diarrhea • Altitude • Respiratory • Motion • First aid
- Women's health • Allergic reaction

KEY POINTS

- The traveler's medical kit is an essential tool for both the novice and expert traveler. Travelers' medical kits are designed to treat travel-related illness and injury and to ensure preexisting medical conditions are managed appropriately.
- Travelers are at increased risk for common gastrointestinal issues during travel, such as infectious diarrhea, constipation, nausea, and/or gastroesophageal reflux disease.
- Respiratory illnesses, usually upper or lower respiratory tract infections, make up approximately 8% of the ailments present in returned international travelers.
- Approximately 12% of travelers experience a travel-related skin condition, such as contact dermatitis from plant toxins, bacterial skin infections, and/or fungal infections, like tinea pedis.
- First aid treatment for minor injuries is essential to all travel medical kits. The complexity ranges from a small, simple case for the urban traveler to a larger, extensive case for wilderness travel.

INTRODUCTION

The traveler's medical kit is an essential tool for both the novice and expert traveler. Its size and complexity depends on the length of travel, travel destination (urban vs remote), activities, and age and health of the traveler. Travelers' medical kits are designed to treat travel-related illness and injury and to ensure preexisting medical conditions are managed appropriately.[1,2] For most travelers, the medical kit provides treatment for common health issues that are acquired abroad and provides peace of mind for the unexpected travel mishap.

Personal Health

All travelers are encouraged to carry documentation of their current health status. Personal health documentation should include the following:

- All allergies (medications, vaccines, foods, toxins)
- Current medications (prescribed and over the counter [OTC])

Department of Pediatrics, University of Washington, Box 354410, Seattle, WA 98195-4410, USA
* Corresponding author.
E-mail address: nhaulman@uw.edu

Med Clin N Am 100 (2016) 261–277
http://dx.doi.org/10.1016/j.mcna.2015.09.007 **medical.theclinics.com**
0025-7125/16/$ – see front matter

- Immunization records
- Current diagnosis list
- Surgical history
- Contact information for health care provider and contact person(s) in case of emergency

Travelers with severe allergies and/or life-threatening health conditions are encouraged to wear a universal medical alert bracelet (www.medicalalert.com). Patients should also review their current health insurance plans and coverage related to international travel before departure. Travelers should consider purchasing a separate policy for medical evacuation coverage.

Prescriptions

All travelers should carry their prescription medications in their original containers in their carry-on luggage and are encouraged to carry an extra supply in a separate location. Travelers may consider carrying a printed and signed prescription for each medication. If additional medications are needed, travelers should be aware that medications obtained in Africa, Asia, and Latin America may be counterfeit drugs. Counterfeit drugs often lack the active drug ingredient, may be expired, and/or may contain harmful additives. Travelers should also be aware of country-specific limitations regarding entrance with medications, such as opiates, cold and cough medications (pseudoephedrine and diphenhydramine), stimulants commonly used for attention-deficit/hyperactivity disorder and attention-deficit disorder, and some antidepressants. In some cases, a physician's letter outlining the reason for treatment may allow the use of such "prohibited" medications. Travelers should contact the embassy and/or consulate of their anticipated destination to ensure there are no restrictions.[1,2]

Resources for counterfeit drugs:

- Centers for Disease Control and Prevention (CDC): www.cdc.gov/Features/CounterfeitDrugs/index.html
- World Health Organization: http://www.who.int/medicines/regulation/ssffc/en/
- Customs and Border Protection

ALLERGIC REACTION

International travelers are at risk for allergic reactions with increased exposure to new insects, new foods, or hidden ingredients in foods due to less-strict labeling laws in the destination country. Examples of in-flight allergic reactions include peanut/tree nut allergies or perfume exposure. Cleaning seats, arm rests, food trays, and door handles with sanitizer wipes can reduce exposure to allergens in flight. As well, travelers may request a nonallergen meal or better yet bring their own food and avoid use of blankets and pillows to reduce in-flight allergen exposure.

Cigarette smoking is more common in countries outside the United States and pollution due to traffic and burning coal is more frequent. Thus, persons with reactive airway disease (RAD) may experience acute breathing problems and should plan accordingly. Persons with a known history of anaphylaxis should carry an epinephrine auto-injector with a minimum of 2 doses for the routine traveler and up to 6 doses for the traveler going to a remote area.[3–5]

The medical kit for allergy prevention and treatment may include the following:

- A short-acting antihistamine: diphenhydramine (Benadryl)
- A long-acting antihistamine: cetirizine (Zyrtec), loratadine (Claritin), fexofenadine (Allegra)

- Fast-acting bronchodilator, such as albuterol for persons with known RAD
- An epinephrine auto-injector preloaded with 0.3 mg 1:1000 epinephrine for persons with known anaphylaxis
- Saline nasal drops to help with congestion secondary to pollutants
- Intranasal steroid sprays for persons with known allergic rhinitis

See **Table 1**, Anaphylaxis, Antihistamine, Inhalers, for dosing, common side effects and contraindications of the previously listed medications.

High-Altitude Medicine

Persons traveling to a high altitude should consider taking the following medications in their medical kit[6–9]:

- Acetazolamide 125-mg tablets
- Dexamethasone 4-mg tablets
- Nifedipine ER 30-mg oral tablet SR 24 HR

See **Table 1**, Acute Mountain Sickness (AMS) Prevention/Treatment, for dosing, common side effects, and contraindications of these medications (see Johnson NJ, Luks AM: High Altitude Medicine, in this issue).

EYE CARE

Common conditions experienced by the traveler include dry eyes, conjunctivitis, corneal abrasions, and other eye injuries. Persons who wear corrective lenses (either glasses or contact lenses) should continue to use their preferred method and carry a backup supply and/or written prescription. Persons using contact lenses should always bring a pair of glasses (with an up-to-date prescription) in the event of eye injury. Persons traveling to high-altitude or sunny destinations should carry UV protection sunglasses or wrap-around eye glasses if exposed to high winds. Air travel and air pollution can cause dry eyes and eye irritation for any traveler. Both can be soothed with lubricating eye drops. Travelers who use either pupillary dilating or constricting eye drops should wear a medical alert bracelet or carry a card in their wallet explaining this condition and which eye has the condition. If going to a very remote area, carrying an eye shield may help protect the eye in the event of a serious eye injury.[10–12] The medical kit should include the following:

- Saline eye drops/ointment
- Contact lens holder
- Spare glasses and contacts
- Topical antibiotic for eye infection/corneal abrasion

See **Table 1**, Antibiotics, for dosing, common side effects, and contraindications of these medications.

FIRST AID

First aid kits can be assembled at home or purchased online, at pharmacies, or at adventure-wilderness stores. The complexity ranges from a small, simple case for the urban traveler to a larger, extensive case for wilderness travel. Each kit should be tailored to the traveler based on health conditions and expected activities. All kits should contain items to treat minor injuries that can occur more frequently abroad due to uneven surfaces, lack of uniformity of step width and height, fewer road hazard signs, and absence

Table 1
Dosing, possible side effects, and contraindications/warnings for medications

Category	Generic Name	Indications	Dosing	Possible Side Effects	Contraindications/ Warnings[a]
AMS Prevention/ Treatment	Acetazolamide 125 mg	AMS prevention	1 po bid starting 24 h before ascent above 10,000 ft; may stop 48 h after arrival at high altitude	Fatigue, frequent urination, paresthesias, diarrhea, taste changes, nausea/ vomiting, rash	Severe allergy to sulfa-based *antibiotics*, severe renal or hepatic disease, glaucoma, BPH
	Dexamethasone 4 mg	AMS Prevention, HACE	1 po tid prn severe AMS or HACE. Descend urgently	Nausea, vomiting, dyspepsia, edema, mood swings, insomnia, anxiety	Diabetes, coexistent serious infection
	Nifedipine ER 30 mg	HAPE	1 po bid for prevention of HAPE	Headache, peripheral edema, dizziness, flushing, nausea, fatigue, palpitations	Uncontrolled hypertension, severe CHF
Anaphylaxis	Epinephrine auto-injector	Anaphylaxis, severe allergic reaction	Preloaded 0.3 mg 1:1000 epinephrine SQ or IM	Palpitations, anxiety, hypertension	None if needed for anaphylaxis
Antacid	Calcium Carbonate 500 mg	GERD	1–2 po q 4–6 h	Constipation, headache, nausea, hypercalcemia	Hypercalcemia, active GI bleed
Antibiotics					
Moderate to Severe Travelers' Diarrhea	Ciprofloxacin 500 mg	Treatment of moderate to severe diarrhea	1 po plus 1–2 loperamide bid up to 3 d maximum	Nausea, vomiting, diarrhea, abdominal pain, dizziness, rash, anxiety, tendinopathy	History (hx) of previous tendinopathy or QT prolongation/ dysrhythmia. Age <18 y
	Azithromycin 250 mg		2 po plus 2 loperamide po qd up to 3 d maximum	Nausea, rash, diarrhea, abdominal pain, dizziness, GERD	Hx of QT prolongation/ dysrhythmia
	Rifaximin 200 mg		1 po tid for 3 d, may use with loperamide	Nausea, dizziness, fatigue, edema, headache, abdominal pain, arthralgia, headache, rash	Liver disease, multiple drug interactions

Prolonged worsening respiratory illness	Azithromycin 250 mg	Sinusitis/Bronchitis	2 po day 1, then 1 po days 2–5	Nausea, rash, diarrhea, abdominal pain, dizziness, GERD	Hx of QT prolongation/ dysrhythmia
	Amoxicillin/clavulanate potassium 875 mg/ 125 mg		1 po bid	Diarrhea nausea, rash, urticaria and vaginitis	Hx of cholestatic jaundice, *Clostridium difficile* colitis, allergy to PCN
Eye infection or corneal abrasion	Polymyxin/ trimethoprim drops	Eye infections/Corneal abrasion	1 drop OU tid for 7 d	Burning, pruritus, eyelid edema	Globe perforation
	Erythromycin ointment		1 application 6 times/d for 7 d	Ocular irritation, erythema	
Skin infection	Mupirocin 2%	Wound infection	Apply tid for 7–10 d	Pain, pruritus	—
	Cephalexin 500 mg	Cellulitis	2 tablets po bid × 7–10 d	Rash, itching, NVD, dizziness	Risk with PCN allergic patient
	Trimethoprim/ sulfamethoxazole 160/800	MRSA	1 po bid for 7–10 d	Rash, itching, fatigue, headache nausea/ vomiting, diarrhea	Rare: Steven's Johnson
UTI	Ciprofloxacin 250 mg	Female UTI	1 po bid for 3 d	See above under TD treatment	
	Nitrofurantoin100 mg		1 po bid for 7 d	Nausea, vomiting, anorexia, abdominal pain, diarrhea, dizziness, headache, fatigue	Renal disease, severe dehydration, 32–42 wk pregnancy
	Trimethoprim/ sulfamethoxazole 160/800		1 po bid for 3 d	See above under Skin infection	
Antifungal	Fluconazole 150 mg	Yeast vaginitis	1 po; may repeat in 72 h if needed	Nausea, headache, rash, vomiting, abdominal pain, diarrhea, dyspepsia, dizziness	Active dysrhythmia
	Miconazole, clotrimazole and terconazole creams		100 mg PV qhs × 7 d	Vulvovaginal burning/ itching/swelling, pelvic pain/cramping	Prior allergic reaction
	Clotrimazole 1%, Ketoconazole 2%, Miconazole 2% creams	Tinea pedis/cruris/ corporis	Apply to affected area bid for 3–4 wk	Pruritus, burning, alopecia, xeroderma, angioedema	Prior allergic reaction

(*continued on next page*)

Table 1
(continued)

Category	Generic Name	Indications	Dosing	Possible Side Effects	Contraindications/ Warnings[a]
Antihistamine					
Short-acting H-1	Meclizine 25 mg	Antimotion	1–2 po 60 min before motion, max 6/24 h	Drowsiness, dizziness, headaches constipation, urinary retention, palpitations, hypotension	Glaucoma, BPD
	Dimenhydrinate 50		1–2 po q 6–8 h 60 min before onset of motion		
	Diphenhydramine 25 mg	Allergic reaction, contact dermatitis, hives, motion sickness and insomnia for diphenhydramine	1–2 po q 4–6 h		
Long-acting H-1	Cetirizine 10 mg Loratadine10 mg Fexofenadine 180 mg		1 po qd	Drowsiness, fatigue, headache, pharyngitis, diarrhea	Hepatic and renal impairment
H-2 blocker	Ranitidine 150 mg	GERD	1–2 po qhs	Dizziness, diarrhea, headache	—
Antimotion/Antiemetic	Promethazine 25 mg tab or suppository	Nausea, motion sickness prevention and treatment	1 po or pr q 12 h or 1 h before motion	Drowsiness, dizziness, headaches constipation, urinary retention, palpitations, hypotension	Dystonic reaction, glaucoma, BPH
	Ondansetron 4 mg tab or OTD		1–2 po or sublingual q 8 h		QT prolongation/ dysrhythmia
	Scopolamine patch		1 patch 8 h before motion for 72 h		History of psychosis, glaucoma, BPH
Antiperistaltic agent	Loperamide 2 mg	Diarrhea	Use with TD antibiotic dose or per package instructions	Constipation	Small bowel obstruction Not for use in those < 6 y of age
Antiviral	Oseltamivir 75 mg	Treatment of influenza A and B	1 po bid for 5 d	Nausea, vomiting, headache, psychiatric	Renal disease requires dosing adjustment
Decongestant	Pseudoephedrine 60 mg	Nasal congestion	1 po bid to qid	Palpitations, anxiety, hypertension	Tachydysrhythmia

Diarrhea treatment and prevention	Bismuth subsalicylate 262 mg	Diarrhea treatment and prevention	1–2 po before meal up to qid	Constipation, black tongue, black stool, rhinitis	Allergy to aspirin, current Coumadin, methotrexate or probenecid use, history of renal insufficiency or gout
	Oral rehydration salts	Fluid replacement, diarrhea treatment	Per package instructions	Nausea, vomiting, diarrhea, abdominal pain	Protracted vomiting, worsening diarrhea, ileus, oliguria
	See antibiotic and antiperistaltic sections above				
Emergency contraception	Levonorgestrel 1.5 mg	Postcoital contraceptive	1 po as soon as possible after unprotected intercourse	Menstrual irregularities, nausea, abdominal pain, fatigue, headache, vomiting, breast tenderness, diarrhea	Pregnancy, undiagnosed vaginal bleeding
	Ulipristal 30 mg		1 po as soon as possible after unprotected intercourse		
Fever	Acetaminophen 325 mg	Fever	1–2 po q 6 h	Thrombocytopenia, rash	Liver disease, alcoholics require altered dosing
Pain	Ibuprofen 400 mg	Pain, swelling, sunburn	1–2 po tid	Dyspepsia, bleeding	Renal disease
Inhalers					
Nasal steroids	Multiple	Environmental allergies	1–2 sprays each nostril qd to bid	Epistaxis, anosmia, headache, thrush	Active nasal ulceration
Fast-acting bronchodilator	Albuterol MDI	Allergic reaction, bronchospasm	1–2 puffs q 4–6 h	Nervousness, tremor, palpitations, nausea, dizziness	Tachydysrhythmia
Inhaled corticosteroids	Multiple	Asthma and COPD	1–2 puffs bid	Thrush, cataracts	—

(continued on next page)

Table 1
(continued)

Category	Generic Name	Indications	Dosing	Possible Side Effects	Contraindications/ Warnings[a]
Laxative					
Bulk laxative	Calcium polycarbophil	Constipation	1 po up to qid with water	Abdominal bloating and cramping, flatulence	History of SBO, active rectal bleed/melena, abdominal pain, vomiting
Stool softener	Docusate sodium 100-mg tablets		1 po bid	Diarrhea, abdominal cramping, rash, throat irritation, bitter taste	Diarrhea, abdominal cramping, rash, throat irritation, bitter taste
Proton pump inhibitor	Omeprazole 20 mg	GERD	1–2 po qhs	Headache, abdominal pain, nausea, diarrhea	Hepatic impairment, hypomagnesemia
Sleep aids	See Diphenhydramine in antihistamine section above				
	Melatonin	Insomnia	Dosing according to package insert based on formulation	Abdominal cramping, diarrhea, dizziness, chest pain, confusion, headache, hypotension, pruritus	Pregnancy, coagulation disorder, depression, glaucoma
	Zolpidem		Females, 5 mg po qhs, males 5–10 mg po qhs	Headache, dizziness, back pain, diarrhea, lightheadedness, palpitations, depression	Concurrent alcohol use, severe depression, hepatic impairment
Steroid creams	Hydrocortisone ointment 1% Triamcinolone ointment 0.1%	Contact dermatitis	Apply bid to qid for 10–14 d Apply bid for 10–14 d	Burning, folliculitis, hypopigmentation, skin atrophy, secondary infection	Active bacterial skin infection, large area of open sores

Abbreviations: bid, twice a day; COPD, chronic obstructive pulmonary disease; GERD, gastroesophageal reflux disease; GI, gastrointestinal; IM, intramuscular; po, by mouth; q, every; qd, every day; qid, 4 times a day; tid, 3 times a day; SBO, small bowel obstruction; SQ, subcutaneous; UTI, urinary tract infection.

[a] Allergy or hypersensitivity to the medication in the past or to any component in the formulation is an understood contraindication to taking the medication.

of sidewalks. Also the traveler should prepare for more walking with comfortable shoes and may consider carrying a collapsible walking stick.[11]

In addition to medications discussed in other sections of this article the first aid kit should include the following:

- An ample supply of adhesive strips of varying sizes (waterproof and breathable)
- Antiseptic (chlorhexidine swab) antibacterial/antiseptic or alcohol-based sanitizers
- Elastic bandage 3 inch (Ace wrap) for sprains or for compression
- Disposable examination gloves
- Adhesive tape
- Gauze (4 × 4 inches, 2 × 2 inches, and tube)
- An OTC antibiotic ointment
- Moleskin/molefoam
- A small pair of tweezers that can be used to remove ticks, slivers, and dirt particles from wounds
- Wound glue for minor lacerations
- Thermometer
- Several safety pins to be used as quick repairs for tears in clothing or luggage
- Duct tape for repairs as well as temporary wound closure for larger lacerations
- Scissors
- Ibuprofen for pain
- Acetaminophen for fever
- Sunscreen (see skin section)
- Hand sanitizer liquid or sanitizer wipes
- Masks if traveling to areas with high rates of pollution

Adventure travelers to remote areas will also need to bring the following:

- Splints/triangular bandage
- Syringes and needles
- An OTC dental first aid kit that includes Temparin Max (DenTek) to replace a lost filling/cap/crown/inlay and a topical dental antiseptic/anesthetic, such as eugenol. Teeth that are knocked out should be replaced in the gum tissue as soon as possible.
- QuickClot device (usually gauze, surgical dressing mesh) that is impregnated with kaolin to consider for severe bleeding injuries.

See **Table 1**, Fever/Pain, for drug category, dosing, and common side effects and contraindications of these medications.

GASTROINTESTINAL DISORDERS

Travelers are at increased risk for common gastrointestinal issues during travel, such as infectious diarrhea, constipation, nausea, and/or gastroesophageal reflux disease (GERD). Changes in food intake, level of food and water hygiene, length of time traveling, and individual risks are contributing factors. All travelers should carry self-treatment options for common gastrointestinal conditions. In addition, individuals with severe gastrointestinal conditions, such as inflammatory bowel disease, should be highly selective about safe food and water ingestion and carry self-treatment for disease exacerbations and new infections. Possible items to include in the medical kit are the following:

- ORS (oral rehydration salts)
- Bismuth subsalicylate (Pepto-Bismol) 262 mg

- Loperamide (Imodium) 2 mg
- Azithromycin (Zithromax) 250-mg tablets or
- Ciprofloxacin (Cipro) 500-mg tablets or
- Rifaximin (Xifaxan) 200 mg tablets
- Ondansetron (Zofran) 4 or 8 mg tablets
- Promethazine 25 mg tablets or rectal suppositories
- Calcium carbonate 500 mg (Tums)
- Ranitidine (Zantac) 75 mg
- Omeprazole (Prilosec) 20 mg once a day
- Calcium polycarophil (FiberCon)
- Docusate sodium (Colace) 100-mg tablets

Traveler's Diarrhea Treatment

Diarrhea treatment includes replacing lost fluids with clear liquids and/or ORS, slowing peristalsis (as needed use of loperamide), and/or treatment with antibiotics if diarrhea is moderate to severe. The following should be included in most medical kits:

- ORS
- Bismuth subsalicylate (Pepto-Bismol) 262 mg
- Loperamide
- Antibiotics depending on travel destination and health history

ORS can be purchased as packets worldwide or can be prepared as followed:

- 30 mL (6 teaspoons) sugar, 2.5 mL (0.5 teaspoon) salt in 1 L sterile or filtered water
- *Caution*: hyperkalemia, hypernatremia can occur due to inappropriate preparation of ORS

Bismuth subsalicylate can be used before a questionable meal for diarrhea prevention and for treatment of diarrhea. Loperamide is used in different dosing schedules depending on the severity of the diarrhea. For milder forms of diarrhea, one can follow the package insert, which recommends 2 tablets (4 mg) at onset of diarrhea followed by 1 tablet with each subsequent stool up to 5 maximum in 24 hours. If taking with an antibiotic, loperamide is only used at the same time as the antibiotic is taken to avoid possible constipation and delay in passage of the bacteria.

Other Gastrointestinal Symptoms

Nausea

Nausea can be prevented or treated with ondansetron 4-mg or 8-mg oral or sublingual tablets or Phenergan 25-mg tablets or rectal suppositories.

Gastroesophageal Reflux Disease

GERD can be treated with an antacid such as calcium carbonate (Tums), an H-2 blocker such as ranitidine (Zantac), or for worsening symptoms a proton pump inhibitor such as omeprazole (Prilosec).

Constipation

Constipation can be treated with bulk-forming laxatives such as calcium polycarophil (FiberCon) or stool softeners such as docusate sodium (Colace) 100 mg-tablets.[13–16]

See **Table 1**, Antiemetic, Antihistamine (H2 blocker), Antacid, Laxative and Proton Pump Inhibitor, Diarrhea, Antibiotic, and Antiperistaltic, for dosing, common side effects, and contraindications of these medications.

ARTHROPOD AVOIDANCE

Adventure travelers and travelers to the tropics encounter mosquitoes, flies, ticks, and other insects. Some are merely a nuisance; others are vectors of serious diseases. Strategies to reduce bites include use of repellents for skin and for clothing and use of environmental controls such as bet nets, screens, and burning oils, and use of coils.

Skin repellents are applied directly to exposed skin. Overall efficacy of any of the skin repellents is based on concentration and formulation as well as environmental factors such as humidity, rain, wind, level of personal activity and sweat production, how dense the arthropod population is, and how attractive the traveler is to arthropods.[17]

Insect repellent recommended for a travel kit may include any of the following.

For skin:

- DEET (N,N-diethyl-methylbenzamide) (20%–50%)
- Picaridin (2-[2-hydroxyethyl]-piperidinecarboxylic acid methyl ester) (20%)
- PMD, lemon eucalyptus extract (*p*-Menthane-3,8-diol isomers) (30%–50%)

For clothing:

- 3-phenoxybenzyl (1RS,3RS;1RS,3SR)-3-(2,2-dichlorovinyl)-2,2-dimethyl-cyclopropanecarboxylate (permethrin)

DEET as a lotion (20%–50%) is considered to be the most effective protection against arthropod bites. The duration of action is based on the concentration and formulation. The extended-duration 35% DEET gives 12 hours of protection affording twice-a-day application to protect against both day and evening biting arthropods. DEET should not be applied to clothing or netting; wrist bands with DEET are ineffective.

Twenty percent picaridin (also known as icaridin) comes in a liquid spray requiring more frequent application. Lower concentrations are less effective. Some formulations offer up to 8 hours of protection.

Thirty percent to 50% PMD (lemon eucalyptus extract) may be as effective as DEET. At a concentration of 30%, its duration of action is somewhat shorter than that of DEET or picaridin; it has been found to be effective for 4 to 6 hours against mosquitoes and ticks. Spraying pants, socks, and shoes has been shown to be effective against leech attachment.[18]

Other insect repellents, including citronella, neem, and essential oils are highly volatile and have very short duration of coverage. Given this limitation, they are not recommended for skin protection.

Permethrin (0.5% Solution)

Clothing is either sprayed or soaked in permethrin before travel and at intervals recommended by the manufacturer. Clothing and bed nets impregnated with permethrin can be purchased at adventure and outfitter stores and offer a much longer duration of action than either spraying or soaking.

Burning mosquito coils or use of electric insecticide vapors may kill and/or deter nuisance insects; however, these products have not been shown to prevent arthropod-borne diseases. Inhaling the fumes has been associated with lung cancer. These products are not recommended for disease prevention, inside use, or long-term exposure.

For more details on insect avoidance and prevention, consult the article on personal protection measures (see Alpern JD, Dunlop SJ, Dolan BJ, et al: Personal Protection Measures Against Mosquitoes, Ticks, and Other Arthropods, in this issue).[17,18]

MOTION SICKNESS

Motion sickness is a condition that occurs with real or perceived motion. The degree experienced by any individual is person-dependent; some require very little stimulation, others may be somewhat immune to the effects of motion.[19,20] During travel abroad, motion sickness can occur during boat travel; prolonged car, bus, or train rides; or during activities such as riding on centripetal carnival rides, rock climbing, or bungee jumping.

The symptoms of motion sickness (malaise, warmth, sweating, nausea, and dizziness) occur when the brain receives incongruent signals from the vestibular, visual, and proprioceptive systems. Prolonged motion sickness may result in drowsiness, lack of concentration, and apathy. Receptors involved in motion sickness include cholinergic, sympathomimetic and dopaminergic receptors. Blocking these receptors with anticholinergics has been the mainstay of treatment.[19] They can be used as prevention as well as treatment of motion sickness.

In addition to medications, visualization techniques, such as focusing on a distant object or the horizon, lying flat on a boat, practiced diaphragmatic breathing, and taking control of driving or steering or sitting in the front seat of a car may lessen or alleviate the symptoms of motion sickness.[21]

Medications that prevent and treat motion sickness include the following:

- Antihistamines
- Scopolamine
- Promethazine 25 mg (Phenergan)
- Ondansetron 4 to 8 mg (Zofran)

Antihistamines, such as dimenhydrinate (Dramamine), diphenhydramine (Benadryl), and meclizine (Bonine) are effective for prevention and treatment of motion sickness.

Scopolamine patches are felt to be the most effective medication for motion sickness prevention. To be effective, however, the patch needs to be applied post auricular at least 4 hours before anticipated motion. The most common reason for discontinuing use is a local rash.

Promethazine is a phenothiazine and an anticholinergic medication and has the potential to cause a dystonic reaction. It can be taken orally or as a rectal suppository.

Ondansetron is a well-tolerated antiemetic and has the added benefit of coming in sublingual tablets.

See **Table 1**, Antihistamine, Antimotion/Antiemetic dosing, for common side effects and contraindications of these medications.

MALARIA PREVENTION

Malaria is the most significant worldwide arthropod-borne disease that can be prevented with medication and insect precautions. The malaria-infected female *Anopheles* mosquito bites from dusk to dawn. Staying indoors during the evening hours, wearing long sleeves and long pants, sleeping under mosquito nets, and using insecticides and repellents can lessen exposure.[22]

Chemoprophylaxis medications remain the mainstay of prevention for persons traveling to known malaria risk areas. The following medications are used for malaria prophylaxis:

- Chloroquine or hydroxychloroquine (for chloroquine-sensitive malaria only)
- Mefloquine

- Doxycycline
- Atovaqoune-Proguanil

For more details on chemoprophylaxis therapy and specific indications for use and geographic utility of these medications, consult the article on malaria prevention (see Hahn WO, Pottinger PS: Malaria in the Traveler: How to Manage Before Departure and Evaluate Upon Return, in this issue).

RESPIRATORY ILLNESS

Upper and lower respiratory tract infections make up approximately 8% of the ailments present in returned international travelers.[23] These illnesses can range from upper respiratory infections to bronchitis/pneumonia and influenzalike illness and are usually transmitted by droplet infection or direct contact. Pathogens include viruses, bacteria, and, rarely, fungi and parasites. High-risk patients (those with chronic obstructive pulmonary disease or asthma, or who are immune-suppressed) may benefit from carrying a broad-spectrum antibiotic in the case of a prolonged respiratory illness. Concern over the growing prevalence of antibiotic resistance dictates judicious use of this practice.[24]

The medical kit for treatment of respiratory symptoms and illness includes the following:

- Nasal saline drops
- Pseudoephedrine (Sudafed)
- Intranasal steroids spray
- Antihistamines
- Albuterol
- Inhaled steroid
- Antibiotics (azithromycin, amoxicillin, or amoxicillin clavulanate)
- Oseltamivir (Tamiflu) if traveling during influenza season and is at high risk

See **Table 1**, Antihistamine, Antibiotics, Antiviral, Decongestants, and Inhalers, for dosing, common side effects, and contraindications of these medications.

SLEEP DISRUPTION/JET LAG

Sleep disruption is common in travelers due to rapid changes in time zones with air travel. This condition is caused by physiologic changes in an individual's circadian rhythm. Treatment recommendations aim to help the traveler adjust more quickly to a new time zone and are not recommended for sleep on airplanes.[22]

Options include the following:

- Diphenhydramine (Tylenol PM, Sominex, Unisom)
- N-acetyl-5-methoxy tryptamine (Melatonin)
- Zolpidem (Ambien)

See **Table 1**, Antihistamine, Sleep Aids, for dosing, common side effects and contraindications of these medications.

SKIN CONCERNS

Approximately 12% of travelers experience a travel-related skin condition, such as contact dermatitis from plant toxins, bacterial skin infections, and/or fungal infections, for example, tinea pedis. Travelers are encouraged to bring treatments for common skin issues, as well as treatments for exacerbations of chronic skin concerns.

Information regarding safe sunscreen use is also included in this section. The medical kit may include the following:

- Fungal infections (clortrimazole, ketonconazole, miconazole creams)
- Bacterial skin infections (cephalexin, mupirocin, trimethoprim/sulfamethoxazole)
- Contact dermatitis (cetirizine, diphenhydramine, hydrocortisone 1% or triamcinolone ointment 0.1%, Zanfel)
- Sunscreens (zinc oxide, titanium dioxide, avobenzone, oxybenzone, dioxybenzone, or sulsiobenzone)

Zanfel

Zanfel removes urishiol (oil found on plants such as poison ivy, oak, and sumac and others) by binding with it to create an aggregate cluster. This can then be easily washed away with water. Zanfel should be applied to affected skin as soon as possible after exposure and apply until itching resolves.

Sunscreen

Many travelers are at increased risk due to the damaging rays of the sun through travel to the tropics, high elevation, and travel during the summer. Broad-spectrum sunscreens that block both UVA and UVB rays are the most effective. Sunburn is primarily caused by UVB. Both UVB and UVA can cause sunburn, skin cancer, and premature skin aging.

Broad-spectrum sunscreen: minimum SPF of 15 to maximum SPF of 50+. Active ingredients include zinc oxide, titanium dioxide, avobenzone, oxybenzone, dioxybenzone, or sulsiobenzone. Apply to skin 15 minutes before exposure.

See **Table 1**, Antibiotics, Antifungal, Antihistamines, for drug category, dosing, and common side effects and contraindications of these medications.

SEXUAL HEALTH

Historically, foreign travel is a known contributor to increased sexual activity. Travelers with increased numbers of sexual partners and unprotected sex have an increased risk for sexually transmitted infections (STIs). Approximately 20% of international travelers experience casual sex with travel and about half of these individuals have unprotected intercourse. Travelers are encouraged to have a consistent form of contraception and to always use condoms for prevention of STIs. Risk factors for having a new sexual partner with travel include length of travel, young age, male gender, single status, travel alone, previous history of multiple sexual partners, and/or a previous STI history.[25]

WOMEN'S HEALTH

Statistics show that women who are single and traveling alone are more likely to have a new sexual partner and/or unprotected intercourse. These women are at increased risk for STIs, unwanted pregnancy, induced abortion, and pelvic inflammatory disease. Women are encouraged to have a contraceptive plan before travel, receive the HPV vaccine before travel (if age appropriate) and to always use condoms. The following are options to include in a medical kit for women:

- Yeast vaginitis self-treatment: topical azoles (miconazole, clotrimazole, and terconazole) and oral fluconazole (Diflucan)
- Contraception

- Emergency contraception (EC; Ella and Plan B One-Step)
- Urinary tract infection (UTI) self-treatment (nitrofurantoin, ciprofloxacin, trimethoprim/sulfamethoxazole)

Vaginitis

Women are commonly prescribed self-treatment for a vaginal yeast infection for travel. Major risk factors for yeast vaginitis include use of antibiotics, history of immunosuppression or diabetes, and/or use of contraceptives, such as oral contraceptive pills or intrauterine devices. Options for self-treatment include topical agent and/or oral fluconazole. Most female travelers prefer to carry fluconazole due to the ease of dosing and convenience of size.

Contraception

An increasing number of women traveling for extended trips are considering use of an IUD (intrauterine device) or contraceptive implants (etonogestrel implant systems) rather than oral contraceptive pills (OCPs). Both the IUD (Para Gard, Mirena) and Implantable devices (Nexplanon) are more effective than OCPs and eliminate the need for carrying extra supplies, such as OCP packets. Condoms continue to be a viable, inexpensive contraceptive option for travelers and are important for STI prevention.

Emergency Contraception

In the event of contraceptive failure or sexual violence, many female travelers carry EC. Unfortunately, EC is not available throughout most of the developing world. Female travelers are encouraged to carry a filled prescription for EC which is obtained within the United States before travel.

Options for EC include the following:

- Levonorgestrel (Plan B One-Step) 1.5 mg
- Ulipristal (Ella) 30 mg

Levonorgestrel has maximum efficacy if taken within 72 hours of intercourse, whereas ulipristal can be effective if taken up to 120 hours post coitus.[25–29]

Urinary Tract Infection Treatment

Women at increased risk for UTIs may consider carrying a self-treatment dose of antibiotics. Current guidelines indicate that women are very effective at self-diagnosis of a UTI. In addition, women understand symptoms to suggest a worsening infection (fever, vomiting, flank or abdominal pain) and need for additional evaluation.

- Nitrofurantoin (Macrobid) 100 mg
- Trimethoprim/sulfamethoxazole (Bactrim DS, Septra DS) 160/800 mg
- Ciprofloxacin (Cipro) 250 mg

See **Table 1**, Antibiotics, Antifungal, Emergency Contraception, for dosing, common side effects and contraindications of these medications.

Medical Kits Available for Purchase

American Red Cross www.redcrossstore.org

Adventure Medical kits

Chinook Medical Gear www.chinookmed.com

Wilderness Medicine Outfitters www.wildernessmedicine.com

REFERENCES

1. The yellow book: health information for international travel. Centers for Disease Control and Prevention (CDC). Available at: www.nc.cdc.gov/travel/yellowbook/2014.
2. Harper L, Bettinger J, Dismukes R, et al. Evaluation of the Coca-Cola Company travel health kit. J Travel Med 2002;9:244–6.
3. Barnett J, Botting N, Gowland MH, et al. The strategies that peanut and nut-allergic consumers employ to remain safe when travelling abroad. Clin Transl Allergy 2012;2(12):1–7. Available at: http://www.ctajournal.com/content/2/1/12.
4. Greenhawt M, MacGillivray F, Batty G, et al. International study of risk-mitigating factors and in-flight allergic reactions to peanut and tree nut. J Allergy Clin Immunol Pract 2013;1(2):186–94.
5. Stokes S, Hudson S. Managing anaphylaxis in a jungle environment. Wilderness Environ Med 2012;23:51–5.
6. Luks A. High altitude medicine. University of Washington; 2011. 13th Update on Travel Medicine and Global Health.
7. Auerbach PS. Wilderness medicine. 6th edition. Philadelphia: Mosby Elsevier; 2012.
8. Sven s, Daene M, Dilissen E, et al. Effects of high altitude and cold air exposure on airway inflammation in patients with asthma. Thorax 2013;68:906–13.
9. Pollar A, Murdoch D. The high altitude medicine handbook. 3rd edition. 2003.
10. Morris DS, Mella S, Depla D. Eye problems on expeditions. Travel Med Infect Dis 2013;11:152–8.
11. Kupper T, Rieke B, Neppach K, et al. Health hazards and medical treatment of volunteers aged 18-30 years working in international social projects of non-governmental organizations (NGOs). Travel Med Infect Dis 2014;12(4):385–95.
12. Chen LH, Wilson ME, Davis X, et al. Illness in long-term traveler's visiting geosentinel clinics. Emerg Infect Dis 2009;15(11):1773–82. Available at: www.cdc.gov/EID/content/15/11/1773.htm.
13. Jong E, Sanford C. The travel and tropical medicine manual. 4th edition. Saunders; 2008.
14. Dupont HL, Ericcson CD. Prevention and treatment of traveler's diarrhea. N Engl J Med 1993;328:1821.
15. Intensive Update Course in Clinical Tropical Medicine and Traveler's Health. Sponsored by the American Society of Tropical Medicine and Hygiene (ASTMH). October 27-28, 2009.
16. Eddleston M, Davidson R, Wilkinson R, et al. Oxford, handbook of tropical medicine. Oxford (United Kingdom): Oxford University Press; 2005.
17. Goodyer L, Croft A, Frances S, et al. Expert review of the evidence base for arthropod bite avoidance. J Travel Med 2010;17(3):182–92.
18. Kirton LG. Laboratory and field tests of the effectiveness of the lemon-eucalyptus extract, citriodiol, as a repellent against land leeches of the genus *Haemadipsa* (Haemadipsidae). Ann Trop Med Parasitol 2005;99(7):695–714.
19. Nachum Z, Shupak A, Gordan CR. Transdermal scopolamine for prevention of motion sickness. Clin Pharmacokinet 2006;45(6):543–66.
20. Weerts A, Putcha L, Hoag S, et al. Intranasal scopolamine affects the semicircular canals centrally and peripherally. J Appl Phys 2015;119(3):213–8.
21. Stromberg SE, Russell ME, Carlson CR. Diaphragmatic breathing and its effectiveness for the management of motion sickness. Aerosp Med Hum Perform 2015;86(5):452–7.

22. Leder K, Black J, O'Brien D, et al. Malaria in travelers: a review of GeoSentinel Surveillance Network. Clin Infect Dis 2004;39(8):1104–12.
23. Harvey K, Esposito DH, Han P, et al. Surveillance for travel-related disease – GeoSentinel Surveillance System, United States, 1997-2011. MMWR Surveill Summ 2013;62(3):1–23.
24. Korzeniewski K, Nitsch-Osuch A, Lass A, et al. Respiratory infections in travelers from the tropics. Adv Exp Med Biol 2015;848:75–82.
25. Sack RL. Clinical practice. Jet lag. N Engl J Med 2010;362(5):440–7.
26. Ward B. Travel and sexually transmitted infections. J Travel Med 2006;12(5):300–17.
27. Vicancos R, Abubakar I, Hunter P. Foreign travel associated with increased sexual risk taking, alcohol, and drug use amount UK university students: a cohort study. Int J STD AIDS 2010;21:46–51.
28. Glasier AF, Cameron ST, Fine PM, et al. Ulipristal acetate versus levonorgestrel for emergency contraception: a randomised n-inferiority trial and meta-analysis. Lancet 2010;375(9714):555–62.
29. Snow SE, Melilo SN, Jarvis CI. Ulipristal acetate for emergency contraception. Ann Pharmacother 2011;45(6):780–6.

Care for the Health Care Provider

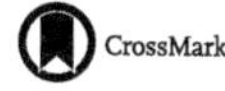

Sharon Brown Kunin, DO, MS[a,*], David Mitchell Kanze, DO[b]

KEYWORDS

• Travel medicine • Global health care provider • Pretravel care • Global health
• Infectious disease prevention • International travel health

KEY POINTS

- Prevention is better than cure.
- The importance of pretravel care for the health care provider.
- The importance of adherence to travel recommendations.
- The importance of vaccinations and PEP.
- The importance of knowing where to access travel health information.

Prevention is better than cure.
—Desiderius Erasmus

INTRODUCTION

The foundation of pretravel care for the health care provider (HCP) begins with prevention. This includes a travel risk assessment and thorough inventory review by a primary care physician, who is versed in travel medicine, or a travel medicine expert. Many travel pitfalls and illnesses can be prevented when appropriate destination-specific travel advice, chemoprophylaxis, and vaccinations are instituted. International travel provides an amazing opportunity to explore new cultures and embark on new adventures, but unfortunately sometimes it also involves introduction to new diseases. With all the excitement, as many as 90% of travelers often forget sage advice and indulge in unsafe food and drink within several days of arrival,[1] and many report illnesses while abroad,[2–4] most of which are caused by gastrointestinal and febrile illness.

Tourist travelers are projected to reach 1 billion,[3] and US residents make more than 61 million trips outside the country.[5] Tourists represent the majority of travelers (38%), and the next largest group is missionary/volunteer/research aide workers (24%–25%).[5]

[a] Department of Family Medicine, University of Washington, Seattle, WA, USA; [b] Family Medicine/Osteopathic Manipulative Treatment Residency Program, Skagit Regional Health, 819 South 13th Street, Mount Vernon, WA 98274, USA
* Corresponding author. PGY 3 Skagit Regional Health Family Medicine and Osteopathic Manipulative Treatment Residency Program, 1415 East Kincaid Street, Mount Vernon, WA 98273.
E-mail address: sbkunin@gmail.com

Med Clin N Am 100 (2016) 279–288
http://dx.doi.org/10.1016/j.mcna.2015.07.012 **medical.theclinics.com**

Worldwide, 8% to 20% of travelers from industrialized to developing countries report becoming ill enough to seek health care during or after travel.[4–7] Many others experience health problems that often go unreported.[1,8] Unfortunately, only 40% to 50% of travelers seek travel health advice, and only 50% to 60% of travelers are fully compliant with malaria chemoprophylaxis.[3,9] Humanitarian service workers often face increased risks of illness and injury based on the nature of their work and travel destinations.[10,11]

Addressing the health care needs of the global HCP is essential, and this process begins with a pretravel risk assessment[12] by an expert.[4,13–15] The global HCP should not attempt to do this for himself or herself, as something is frequently left out. A travel medicine specialist is recommended, particularly for high-risk groups such as health care providers, as they are inevitably at greater health risk than regular travelers.[10,11,16] The global HCP's own medical needs must be taken into account before planning a global mission. HCPs must be aware of all medical conditions that may be encountered in the countries to be visited and medications required to prevent complications while abroad. They must do everything in their power in order to prevent becoming a patient. This includes vaccinations, malarial prophylaxis (if required), and management of their own chronic health conditions. The travel risk assessment of each individual provider, and traveler, should yield an individualized pretravel education plan that includes the details listed previously. Having an emergency plan, evacuation insurance, in-country embassy information, and other critical resources readily available is essential to the success of medical missions.

The essential pretravel inventory includes all the destinations, length of stay, logistical arrangements, type of lodging, food and water supply, medical kit, team members, personal medical needs, and the needs of the community the HCP is going to serve. This inventory must be fluid. Pretravel care and risk assessment based on destination-specific health risks are essential. In addition, having key resources (books and technology) at one's fingertips can really help (**Table 1**).[17] This article will help demonstrate the medical requirements and recommendations for such planning so that the mission is an unmitigated success for the provider and the people in need.

PREVENTING MORBIDITY AND MORTALITY

The GeoSentinel Surveillance System is the largest repository of provider-based data on travel-related illness. Data collected from September 1997 to December 2011 on 141,789 ill returned travelers showed fewer than half (44%) reported having had a pretravel visit with a health care provider. The most common diagnostic groupings were acute diarrhea (22%), nondiarrheal gastrointestinal illness (15%), febrile/systemic illness (14%), and dermatologic conditions (12%).[4] Gastrointestinal diagnoses were most frequent, suggesting that US travelers might be exposed to unsafe food and water while traveling internationally. The most common febrile/systemic diagnosis was *Plasmodium falciparum* malaria, suggesting that some US travelers to malarial areas are not receiving or using proper malaria chemoprophylaxis or mosquito bite avoidance measures. Similar findings were apparent in data collected on 42,173 ill returned travelers seen between 2007 and 2011, showing gastrointestinal (34.0%), febrile (23.3%), and dermatologic (19.5%) diseases. Only 40.5% of all ill travelers reported pretravel medical visits.[3] In a prospective study of 784 travelers, an illness was reported by 64% of travelers, diarrhea being the most common in 46% of travelers, followed by respiratory illness in 26% of travelers, skin disorders in 8% of travelers, acute mountain sickness in 6% of travelers, motion sickness in 5% of travelers, accidents and injuries in 4% of travelers, and isolated febrile episodes in 3% of travelers.[7]

Table 1
Resources for the health care provider

Resource: Web site, APP or Book	Resource Information Provided?
Best Web sites	
CDC www.cdc.gov/travel Excellent resource	CDC Up-to-date health information for travelers • Immunizations • Malaria prevention • Updates on emerging health risks
CDC's "The Yellow Book"—online and in print http://wwwnc.cdc.gov/travel/page/yellowbook-home Excellent resource	CDC health information for international travel resource for physicians with up-to-date information for preparation of travelers—updated every other year • Updated vaccine requirements and recommendations • Diseases related to travel: how to prevent diagnose and treat them • How to prevent and treat other health risks: that is, travelers' diarrhea • Advice for special types of travel (ie, humanitarian aid work and medical tourism)
World Health Organization. http://www.who.int/ith/en International travel and health	International travel and health information page, disease info, vaccines, travel kit checklist, and other information
Applications for one's mobile phone/device: The use of technology can really help!!	
CDC's TravWell application helps one plan for safe and healthy international travel Key features • No data connection needed • Fully customizable to do list and packing list • Emergency services phone numbers	• Destination-specific vaccine recommendations • Checklist of what one need's to do to prepare for travel • Customizable healthy travel packing list • Store travel documents • Keep a record of one's medications and immunizations • Set reminders to get vaccine booster doses or take medicines while traveling
CDC's Can I Eat This App? Key Features – • Access up-to-date recommendations offline • No data connection needed	• This mobile application will tell one whether the food one wants to eat is likely to be safe • This application may end up being an essential part of one's preventive health care in country; Just select the country and answer a few simple questions about what one ise thinking about eating or drinking, and Can I Eat This? will tell whether it is likely to be safe.
Safety essential	
STEP (Smart Traveler Enrollment Program) https://step.state.gov/step/	STEP is a free service to allow US citizens and nationals traveling abroad to enroll their trip with the nearest US embassy or consulate. • Receive important information from the embassy about safety conditions in one's destination country, helping one make informed decisions about travel plans • Help the US Embassy contact one in an emergency, whether natural disaster, civil unrest, or family emergency • Help family and friends get in touch with one in an emergency

(*continued on next page*)

Table 1
(continued)

Resource: Web site, APP or Book	Resource Information Provided?
Other helpful Web sites	
www.state.gov	Travel advisories, consular information
International Society for Travel Medicine www.istm.org	Global travel clinic directory
www.astmh.org	List of travel clinics, country-specific diseases, and other information
www.usembassy.gov.	• Current travel warnings • Country-specific information • Travel alerts
Find a doctor or emergency evacuation information	
Find a doctor Find an air ambulance/medical evacuation company -	http://travel.state.gov/content/passports/english/go/health/doctors.html http://travel.state.gov/content/passports/english/go/health/insurance-providers.html
Books	
The Travel and Tropical Medicine Manual, 5th Edition Christopher A. Sanford, Paul Pottinger, Elaine C. Jong (editors). 2016	Comprehensive resource for health care providers by 2 leading travel medicine experts; great for primary health care providers who counsel patients on travel, infectious disease doctors, and other travel medicine practitioners
Manual of Travel Medicine and Health by Dupont H, Steffen R	Comprehensive resource for HCPs by 2 travel medicine experts

It is essential to know where and how to access critical information.

PRECOUNTRY PLANNING/ADVICE

Careful planning and preparation minimize risks to health and maximize the likelihood of success of a trip/mission/adventure.[18,19] The US Centers for Disease Control and Prevention (CDC) recommends that international travelers seek a pretravel medical consultation 4 to 6 weeks before travel. This precountry preparation also includes consulting the following Web sites, including the CDC (www.cdc.gov), the Yellow Book link (http://www.cdc.gov/features/yellowbook/), US Department of State (http://travel.state.gov/content/passports/english/passports.html), the Smart Traveler Enrollment Program (https://step.state.gov/step/), and the World Health Organization (www.WHO.org). These Web sites reveal key information about the countries and regions, including government information, religious and traditional medical practices, local healers, currency, customs, laws, and travel warnings. General travel health topics include: arthropod avoidance (DEET [N,N-Diethyl-meta-toluamide], bed nets, clothing), safe food and water, freshwater swimming, safe behavior, and high altitude.[20] (see **Table 1** for more information).

Essential questions to ask prior to travel include (**Table 2**) the following:

- Itinerary. Where and when? What documents do I need?
- Purpose of the trip. Medical mission, disaster relief, other?
- Required/recommended vaccinations
- Traveler's diarrhea management
- Malaria prevention/chemoprophylaxis
- Medical illness/emergency contingencies
- What to pack?

Table 2
Essential questions

What documents do I need?	• Passport (valid for >6 mo)[a] • Foreign visas (if required)[a] • Medical license[a] • Driver's license (for driving and/or back-up identification)[a] • Copies of itinerary and all airline and hotel information[a] • Medical insurance/evacuation insurance card[a] • Trip cancellation insurance[a] • International calling card[a] • Automatic Teller machine (ATM)/credit cards and traveler checks (with serial numbers)[a] • Cash (in new 20s) • Hospital identification badge • A spreadsheet of all medications (quantities, doses, usage) pharmaceutical category (ie,: antibiotic, antifungal, pain relief...) • Letter from one's private provider detailing why each medication is needed • A spreadsheet of all medical supplies including quantities and usages • Written permission from the government of the country one is entering to practice medicine and bring pharmaceuticals into the country (if required) • Emergency contact list/phone tree for the entire team
What vaccinations do I need?	Resource information—travel expert + CDC, WHO and International Society for Travel Medicine (ISTMH) Web sites • Standard vaccinations (ie, tetanus diphtheria, acellular pertussis; measles, mumps, rubella;, hepatitis B) • Country-specific vaccinations (ie, yellow fever, typhoid, Japanese encephalitis)
What type of prophylaxis/ treatment meds do I need?	• Malarial prophylaxis (Malarone, mefloquine, doxycycline, Coartem, chloroquine (many countries with resistance) and primaquine (in some cases) • Diarrheal prophylaxis (not generally recommended), except probiotics • Diarrheal treatment (ciprofloxacin, azithromycin, rifaxamin, PeptoBismal, loperamide)
What type of medicines and supplies does the country, region, community, clinic, mission need/require?	Medication and medical equipment • How much of each—medication, Supplies, equipment? • Can you bring expired medications? • Are you going with nongovernmental organization or governmental sponsor? • Who pays for the medications and supplies? • What type of mission is it? Disaster relief vs building a medical clinic? • Can your hospital/institution help donate money and/ or equipment

[a] 2 copies (1 stored separately from originals, 1 copy for relatives, always good to have someone who knows how to contact a person in an emergency). Pack in carry-on luggage or "Go-Bag" (small bag with essential items that that one can grab and go somewhere quickly [ie, evacuate in case of emergency]).

Health Care Provider Kit and Packing List

HCPs generally need to pack more than the average traveler. They need to be able to provide for themselves, their team, and the community they are serving. This can be particularly difficult if in a remote region or after a disaster.

Items should fit into a lightweight, strong "Go Bag" that can be taken into any location.

Backpacks or rucksacks are easiest for remote locations. Many items must be stowed for air travel.

An appropriate medical kit should be durable, padded, weatherproof, and easy to carry. A field medicine kit for remote expeditions should include: ear plugs, nail clippers, superglue, suture stapler, thermometer, duct tape (many uses), zip ties, adrenaline (envenomations and allergic reactions and antibiotics) (**Table 3**).[21]

IN COUNTRY CARE

Do what you can, with what you have, where you are.
—Theodore Roosevelt

Food and Water Precautions

A leading cause of morbidity among travelers is gastrointestinal disturbance from food- and waterborne diseases. Traveler's diarrhea is the most common disease among travelers, increasing in frequency when food and water precautions are not strictly practiced. Unwashed (or washed in untreated water) fruits and vegetables are often contaminated with fecal bacteria/parasites. General advice about safe foods is "boil it, cook it, peel it, or forget it". Disinfecting the water involves boiling water or heating it to greater than 70°C (160°F) for 30 minutes; this is necessary to kill all enteric pathogens.[20] If the temperature is greater than 85°C (185°F), pathogens are eliminated within a few minutes. Dry foods are usually safe. Raw or undercooked seafood is risky. Salads should be carefully washed in treated water; dairy products should be pasteurized, and fruits should be peeled. Avoid street vendors or cooking sites with flies and without refrigeration.

Water Disinfection

Tap water is often unsafe, and ice cubes carry viable pathogens.[22] Iodine is preferred over chorine. If using iodine tablets, dissolve 1 tablet in 1 L of water. Use 2 tablets for heavily polluted water. If using chlorine, add 3 drops of chlorine solution to each 1 L of water, mix well, and wait 30 minutes before drinking it (to make chlorine solution = mix 3 level tablespoons of bleaching powder in 1 L of water). Potable water is required to lessen the chance of spreading waterborne disease and to have a functioning health care facility. Concerning water filters, reverse osmosis or iodine resin filters are most likely to remove all microorganisms. Collected water can be improved by using commercial filters, or white cotton cloth that has been boiled in soapy water and rinsed thoroughly, or by using an item of clothing, such as a sari, which can help reduce cholera incidence by 48%.[21–25] Solar radiation and UV filters work for clear water only and are less effective with cloudy water.[26]

Needle Sticks and PostExposure Prophylaxis

HCPs are required to bring prophylaxis for needle stick exposures if needles will be utilized during the mission. Pretravel advice begins by discussing prevention of needle sticks. This information should be relayed to every member of the health care team.

Table 3
Health care provider packing list

First aid supplies	• Band-aids • Moleskin • Adhesive tape • Ace bandage • Antiseptic wound cleanser • Alcohol wipes • Sterile dressing • Sutures and needle driver • Dermabond • Gloves • Scissors • Tweezers • Steri-strips • Safety pins • Suture stapler • Duct tape (many uses) • Lubricant eye drops • Sunscreen/insect repellant • Analgesic (eg, ibuprofen) • Insect bite treatment • Thermometer • Stethoscope • Otoscope/ophthalmoscope • Broselow tape for pediatrics	• Prescription medicine • Antimalarials • Antihistamine (Benadryl) • Antinausea (Compazine) • Antidiarrhea (Cipro, Immodium) • Postexposure prophylaxis • Hand sanitizer • Hydrocortisone 1% cream • Lidocaine • Fluconazole • Bacitracin • Dramamine • Tylenol/Advil • Sudafed • Albuterol inhaler • Prednisone • Nasal decongestant • Oral rehydration salts • Sunscreen • Spare eyeglasses/contacts • Personal protective equip • Shampoo and conditioner • Toilet paper and wipes
Gear	• Proper clothing and footwear • Permethrin-treated bed net and clothing • Swiss Army knife • Leatherman/multitool • Zip ties • Headlamp/flashlight • Water bottle • Water purifier and iodine tablets • Sleeping bag/sheet • Sunglasses/hat • High energy, nonperishable food • Matches (wind/waterproof) • Earplugs	• Field/wilderness medicine book • Google Translate or Canopy • Candles • Luggage locks • Alarm clock • Bandana/scarf • Clothesline • Laundry detergent • Ziploc bags • Translation book • Sink stopper • Sewing kit • Quick dry travel towels
Electronics	• Laptop and power cord • Flash drive • Satellite phone (if available) • Unlocked cell phone + charger • Electrical adapters • Extra batteries	• iPod/Kindle/IPad + charger • Skype headset • Camera + extra batteries • Phone adapters • Surge protector • Global positioning system
Documents	• Passport and visa • Embassy phone numbers • Evacuation Information	• Medical insurance • ATM/credit cards • Cash (in new 20s)

Data from World Health Organization. Medical kit and toilet items. Available at: http://www.who.int/ith/precautions/medical_kit/en/. Accessed July 28, 2015; and Massachusetts General Hospital – Center for Global Health. Center for Global Health Master Packing List. Available at: https://www.mghcgh.org/assets/files/disaster/CGH_Master_Packing_list.pdf. Accessed July 28, 2015.

Needle sticks occur more frequently in unknown work environments, crowded places, and in hurried treatment scenarios.[27] It is advisable to create sharps containers out of hard plastic or metal containers such as tin cans, stock pharmaceutical bottles, or glass bottles if a traditional sharps container is not available.

HCPs should be aware of the epidemiology/diseases of the region(s) to help dictate the type of postexposure prophylaxis. Prophylaxis should be on hand for human immunodeficiency virus (HIV), hepatitis B virus (HBV), and other bloodborne pathogens. One particular disease to note is malaria, because the risk of needle stick transmission may be even higher than that of HIV or hepatitis and is potentially fatal.[28]

In the event that a needle stick occurs, HCPs need to take a complete history from source patient to include the chief and presenting complaints, region/country of origin, and a blood sample for HIV and other testing. Needle stick wounds should be thoroughly cleansed with warm (if available) water and soap. Utilization of caustic agents is not recommended.[29] The HCP patient should be provided with a clear treatment plan to include medications and follow-up in country and back at home.

Postexposure prophylaxis (PEP) medication regimens for HIV should be started as soon as possible and continued for 4 weeks. HIV has a very low risk of transmission (0.3%) but is the most frightening. Regimens should contain 3 (or more) antiretroviral drugs. Expert consultation is recommended, as well as close follow-up that includes counseling, baseline and follow-up HIV testing (up to 4–6 months after exposure), and monitoring for drug toxicity.[29]

A commonly used regimen is

Tenofovir 300 mg + emtricitabine 200 mg: 1 tablet/d

and

Raltegravir: 400 mg tablet twice daily

× 28 days

HBV is highly transmissible via needle sticks. The best prophylaxis for HBV is receiving the HBV vaccination series prior to leaving, which reduces the risk of transmission by 90%. If the exposed person has received the hepatitis B vaccine series, and subsequent testing has been conducted to ensure that the vaccine was effective (Hepatitis surface antibody level of at least 10 IU/L), then no specific treatment is recommended after a bloodborne exposure.

If the source patient is hepatitis B surface antigen (HBsAg) positive, and the exposed patient has had the hepatitis B vaccine series but not subsequent testing for antibody level, then the exposed person should receive a single dose of hepatitis B vaccine.

If the exposed person has not had the hepatitis B vaccines series, then he or she should receive hepatitis B immune globulin (HBIG); additionally, the regular hepatitis B vaccines should be initiated.

Hepatitis C virus (HCV) is another virus that is transmissible via needle stick. The transmission rate is low, however (1.8%). There is no prophylaxis to HCV infection, and approximately one-fifth of infections clear on their own. Treatment should be given to any person who has positive HCV titers 12 weeks after exposure.[28]

Special Conditions

HCPs must take inventory of endemic disease in a given location, including: viral hemorrhagic fevers (eg, Marburg, ebola), drug-resistant tuberculosis, and severe respiratory viral infections. All HCPs should follow needle stick injuries, especially if they have a fever in the weeks following.[30]

FUTURE CONSIDERATIONS/SUMMARY

Pretravel and in-country care of the HCP is an essential component to the success of any global health mission. HCPs need to take an active role in preparing for their medical mission Practitioners must work to prevent travel-related illness and mitigate the risk of infectious disease transmission so as to optimize success of global health service to individuals and communities desperately in need. Health care providers who travel to resource-limited settings remain an understudied travel population.[10,30] Care for the HCP is an area that deserves more attention and research, so as to maximize targeted preventive efforts, and it is hoped that this article inspires others to further study how to best protect health care providers and reduce their risk of illness and injury.

REFERENCES

1. Steffen R, deBernardis C, Banos A. Travel epidemiology—a global perspective. Int J Antimicrob Agents 2003;21(2):89–95.
2. Freedman DO, Weld LH, Kozarsky PE, et al. Spectrum of disease and relation to place of exposure among ill returned travelers. N Engl J Med 2006;354(2):119–30.
3. Leder K, Torresi J, Libman MD, et al. GeoSentinel surveillance of illness in returned travelers, 2007–2011. Ann Intern Med 2013;156:456–68.
4. Harvey K, Esposito DH, Han P, et al. Surveillance for travel-related disease—GeoSentinel Surveillance System, United States, 1997–2011. MMWR Surveill Summ 2013;62:1–23.
5. Hagmann SH, Han PV, Stauffer WM, et al. Travel-associated disease among US residents visiting US GeoSentinel clinics after return from international travel. Fam Pract 2014;31(6):678–87.
6. Steffen R, Rickenbach M, Wilhelm U, et al. Health problems after travel to developing countries. J Infect Dis 1987;156(1):84–91.
7. Hill DR. Health problems in a large cohort of Americans traveling to developing countries. J Travel Med 2000;7(5):259–66.
8. Hill DR, Ericsson CD, Pearson RD, et al. The practice of travel medicine: guidelines by the Infectious Diseases Society of America. Clin Infect Dis 2006;43(12): 1499–539.
9. Chen LH, Keyston JS. New strategies for the prevention of malaria in travelers. Infect Dis Clin North Am 2005;19(1):185–210.
10. Stoney RJ, Jentes ES, Sotir MJ, et al, Global TravEpiNet Consortium. Pre-travel preparation of US travelers going abroad to provide humanitarian service, Global Trav Epi Net 2009–2011. Am J Trop Med Hyg 2014;90(3):553–9.
11. LaRocque RC, Rao SR, Lee J, et al, Global TravEpiNet Consortium. Demographics, travel destinations and pre-travel health care among U.S. international travelers: analysis of the global TravEpiNet surveillance network. Clin Infect Dis 2011;54(4):455–62.
12. Bazemore A, Huntington M. The pretravel consultation. Am Fam Physician 2009; 80(6):583–90.
13. Bender J, Sellman J. Zoonotic Infections in travelers to the Tropics. Prim Care 2002;29:907–29.
14. Reed JM, McIntosh IB, Powers K. Travel Illness and the family practitioner: a retrospective assessment of travel-induced illness in general practice and the effect of a travel illness clinic. J Travel Med 1994;1(4):192–8.

15. Ryan E, Kain K. Health advice and immunizations for travelers. N Engl J Med 2000;342:1716–25.
16. CDC. Travelers' health: see a doctor before you travel. Atlanta (GA): US Department of Health and Human Services; CDC; 2011. Available at: http://wwwnc.cdc.gov/travel/page/see-doctor. Accessed June 28, 2015.
17. Huntzinger A. Practice guidelines: IDSA releases guidelines on travel medicine. Am Fam Physician 2007;75(11):1712–5.
18. CDC. The yellow book. Atlanta (GA): US Department of Health and Human Services; CDC; 2015. Available at: http://wwwnc.cdc.gov/travel/page/yellowbook-home. Accessed June 28, 2015.
19. Schwartz B, LaRocque R, Ryan R. Travel medicine. Ann Intern Med 2012;156(11):ITC6–119.
20. Hill D, Pearson R. Health advice for international travel. Ann Intern Med 1988;108(6):839–52.
21. Iverson K. Improvised medicine. Providing care in extreme environments. The McGraw-Hill Companies. 2012. p. 558–60.
22. Dickens DL, DuPont HL, Johnson PC. Survival of bacterial enteropathogens in the ice of popular drinks. JAMA 1985;253:3141–3.
23. Smith R, Sears S. Blackwell's primary care essentials. Travel medicine. Chapter 5. Blackwell Publishers. 2002. p. 51–3.
24. Young H, Harvey P. Sphere project. Humanitarian charter and minimum standards in disaster response. Disasters 2004;97–104.
25. Colwell RR, Huq A, Islam MS, et al. Reduction of cholera in Bangladeshi villages by simple filtration. Proc Natl Acad Sci U S A 2003;100:1051–5.
26. CDC. Water disinfection. Available at: http://wwwnc.cdc.gov/travel/page/water-disinfection. Accessed June 28, 2015.
27. Trim JC, Elliott TS. A review of sharps injuries and preventative strategies. J Hosp Infect 2003;53:237–42.
28. Tarantola A, Abiteboul D, Rachlinec A. Infection risks following accidental exposure to blood or body fluids in health care workers: a review of pathogens transmitted in published cases. Am J Infect Control 2006;34:367–75.
29. Kuhar D, Henderson D, Struble K, et al. Updated U.S. Public Health Service guidelines for the management of occupational exposures to HIV and recommendations for post-exposure prophylaxis. CDC; 2013. http://stacks.cdc.gov/view/cdc/20711.
30. Kortepeter MG, Seaworth B, Tasker S, et al. Health care workers and researchers traveling to developing-world clinical settings: disease transmission risk and mitigation. Clin Infect Dis 2010;51:1298–305.

Malaria in the Traveler

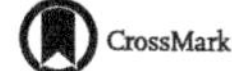

How to Manage Before Departure and Evaluate Upon Return

William O. Hahn, MD*, Paul S. Pottinger, MD, DTM&H, FIDSA

KEYWORDS

• Malaria • Prevention • Chemoprophylaxis • *Plasmodium* • Fever in returning traveler

KEY POINTS

- Medications for malaria chemoprophylaxis work well, and choice of agent is largely dependent on cost and side effects.
- There can be a long lag between acquisition of the malaria parasite and development of disease (months).
- Cyclic fevers are not characteristic of malaria, and many patients present with gastrointestinal disease.
- Rapid diagnostic tests are as sensitive as classic blood smears but do not depend on experienced microscopists.
- In patients from nonendemic areas who return with malaria, it should be treated as a sepsis syndrome.

OVERVIEW

This article familiarizes health care providers with the prevention, diagnosis, and treatment of malaria, with specific focus on patients from nonendemic areas who plan to travel for a limited time to an area with risk of malaria transmission.

Providers must understand malaria, because it is a disease estimated to kill approximately 600,000 people per year worldwide. Despite public health interventions that have reduced the global burden of morbidity and mortality, it remains highly prevalent throughout much of the world. For the general practitioner, it is important to recognize the clinical manifestations of malaria because it is the most common cause of fever in returning travelers[1] and one of the few conditions that can kill patients rapidly if mismanaged. In 2012, approximately 2000 cases were seen in the United States,

Division of Allergy and Infectious Diseases, Department of Medicine, University of Washington, 850 Republican Avenue, Seattle, WA 98109, USA

* Corresponding author. Division of Allergy and Infectious Disease, Box 356423, 1959 Northeast Pacific Street, Seattle, WA 98104.

E-mail address: willhahn@uw.edu

Med Clin N Am 100 (2016) 289–302

http://dx.doi.org/10.1016/j.mcna.2015.09.008 **medical.theclinics.com**

0025-7125/16/$ – see front matter

including 6 preventable deaths.[2] After reading this article, the authors hope that readers will be able to prevent such needless loss of life.

MALARIA

Malaria is an infection caused by any of 5 species of the *Plasmodium* parasite: *P falciparum*, *P vivax*, *P ovale*, *P malariae*, and *P knowlesi* (**Fig. 1**). These single-celled eukaryotic organisms are transmitted to humans by the bite of an *Anopheles* mosquito. Within minutes of the bite, parasites enter the liver, where they develop and multiply asymptomatically. After 10 to 14 days, parasites leave the liver and enter

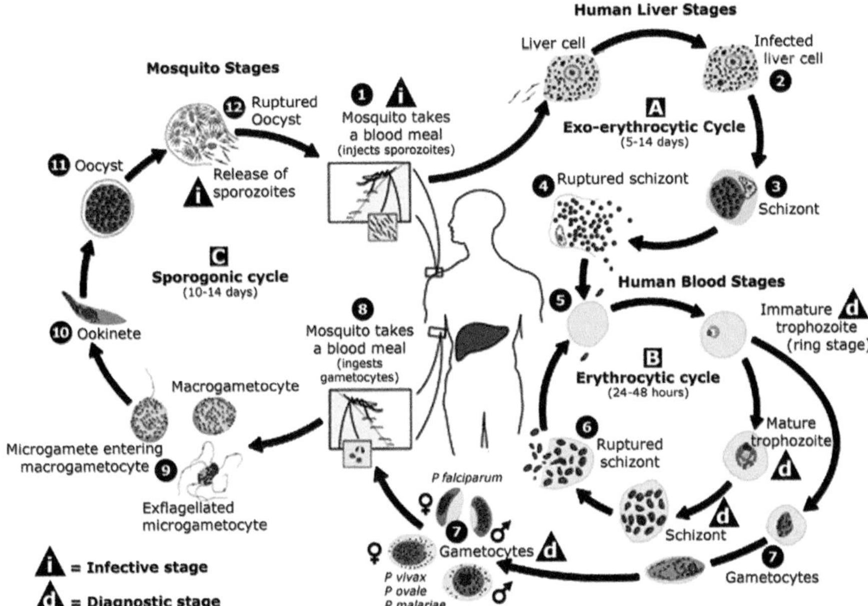

Fig. 1. Malaria life cycle. The malaria parasite life cycle involves 2 hosts. During a blood meal, a malaria-infected female *Anopheles* mosquito inoculates sporozoites into the human host (1). Sporozoites infect liver cells (2) and mature into schizonts (3), which rupture and release merozoites (4). (In *P vivax* and *P ovale*, a dormant stage [hypnozoites] can persist in the liver and cause relapses by invading the bloodstream weeks, or even years, later.) After this initial replication in the liver (exoerythrocytic schizogony [A]), the parasites undergo asexual multiplication in the erythrocytes (erythrocytic schizogony [B]). Merozoites infect red blood cells (5). The ring stage trophozoites mature into schizonts, which rupture, releasing merozoites (6). Some parasites differentiate into sexual erythrocytic stages (gametocytes) (7). Blood-stage parasites are responsible for the clinical manifestations of the disease. The gametocytes, male (microgametocytes) and female (macrogametocytes), are ingested by an *Anopheles* mosquito during a blood meal (8). The parasites' multiplication in the mosquito is known as the sporogonic cycle (C). While in the mosquito's stomach, the microgametes penetrate the macrogametes generating zygotes (9). The zygotes in turn become motile and elongated (ookinetes) (10), which invade the midgut wall of the mosquito where they develop into oocysts (11). The oocysts grow, rupture, and release sporozoites (12), which make their way to the mosquito's salivary glands. Inoculation of the sporozoites (1) into a new human host perpetuates the malaria life cycle. (*From* Centers for Disease Control and Prevention. About malaria. Available at: http://www.cdc.gov/malaria/about/biology/. Accessed August 26, 2015.)

the bloodstream, rapidly invading erythrocytes to feed on hemoglobin, multiply, and, after 2 to 3 days, erupt from the diseased cell to invade new erythrocytes. It is this erythrocytic phase of plasmodium life cycle that is responsible for clinical illness.

In cases of *P vivax* and *P ovale*, some parasites may enter a dormant phase in the liver, which may reactivate months after initial reinfection. These hypnozoites require special treatment.

The plasmodium life cycle is completed when sexual forms of the parasites (gametocytes) are ingested by another *Anopheles* mosquito, allowing them to mate and develop within the insect.

PREVENTION: 4 STEPS TO SUCCESS

No vaccine for malaria prevention currently exists for travelers; exciting developments have taken place in the past decade, demonstrating at least partial protection of a live attenuated vaccine when administered to children living in highly endemic areas. This vaccine is not, however, approved or available for other patient groups. Thus, health care providers should be adept at a multipronged prevention strategy: determine the malaria risk, counsel on mosquito avoidance techniques, prescribe chemoprophylaxis, and educate on warning signs of malaria.

Step 1: Determine Whether a Patient Is at Risk of Malaria

Geographic risk assessment

There are several publicly available resources that can assist in determining whether travel to a particular area is associated with the risk of developing malaria. Foremost is the Centers for Disease Control and Prevention Web site (http://www.cdc.gov/malaria). There are also proprietary databases, such as the Travax Web site (http://www.travax.com), which provide information regarding the current rate of malaria in a particular locales. In general, malaria is not endemic in areas above 3300 m (10,800 ft). Nevertheless, because malaria can be fulminant in non–semi-immune populations, providers should err on the side of offering both advice and chemotherapy if the risk cannot be adequately described. In general, all patients traveling to sub-Saharan Africa are at risk, unless their journey is exclusively to highlands, such as Mount Kilimanjaro; the bulk of imported cases in the United States originate in Africa.[3]

Further complicating travel advice, acquisition of malaria in and around airports is a well-described phenomenon.[4] Travelers, however, who merely change planes or lay over in an airport in malarious regions are generally thought at low risk of infection.

The risk of malaria may rise and fall in a given region based on the season of travel, with highest risk after sustained rains that fill pools with water where mosquitoes breed. In most endemic regions, however, some risk persists year-round, and the time of travel during the dry season does not preclude the need for prevention measures.

On the other hand, real progress has been achieved in certain areas, where the risk of malaria is now negligible compared with years gone by. Whether this has happened due to mosquito control programs or climate change—or both—varies from case to case. Regardless, it is worth consulting an up-to-date resource if providers are not familiar with a particular itinerary, because malaria prophylaxis may no longer be required.

Host risk assessment

Malaria can happen to any patient, even if hailing from an endemic area or having had malaria before, because the semi-immune state wanes within months after exposure ceases. But some patients seem exceptionally susceptible to malaria and deserve special counseling. The strongest association is with HIV/AIDS, where frequency of malaria episodes rises as CD4 counts fall.[5] Patients who have HIV should be advised that they are at higher risk of malaria acquisition, although if they have a high CD4 count and good virologic control, the magnitude of the risk is unknown and probably similar to that in patients without HIV. Trimethoprim/sulfamethoxazole is not adequate malaria prophylaxis in patients traveling to Africa (discussed later).

Asplenia is another well-described risk factor for development of malaria. Patients from an endemic area in Malawi who are asplenic from trauma have been demonstrated to have increased risks of clinical malaria and have higher parasite densities with *P falciparum* than age-matched controls.[6] This was from a population with preexisting immunity to malaria. Therefore, the risk of severe malaria and the clinical course of infection in a naive individual are unknown. Laboratory investigations have demonstrated that both congenitally asplenic and surgically splenectomized mice have a uniformly fatal outcome with malaria infection.[7] Part of any routine counseling prior to departure to a malaria endemic area should include whether a patient is either anatomically or functionally asplenic.

The authors also encourage evaluation of other immunosupression, especially including exposure to medications that deplete or affect the B-cell compartment, such as anti-CD20 antibodies (eg, rituximab). Babesiosis, an analogous intraerythrocytic parasitic disease, is substantially worsened when monoclonal antibodies are given against CD20 (rituximab). In animal studies, B-cell depletion leads to death from infection, and repletion of immune serum has been used therapeutically in malaria infections. Therefore, it is reasonable to assume that any patient with an autoimmune disease on immunomodulatory therapy that affects the B-cell compartment (or $CD4^+$ T-cell subset) is at increased risk for both development of clinical malaria and worse disease outcomes.

Step 2: Counsel on Mosquito Avoidance Techniques

Malaria is a vector-borne illness acquired during the bite of a female *Anopheles* mosquito. An important feature of this mosquito vector is nighttime feeding behavior. This stereotypical behavior makes bed nets an important part of prevention of the disease. Although the efficacy of bed nets in nonendemic populations is unknown, meta-analysis of studies in endemic areas bed nets have demonstrated reduction in the episodes of clinical malaria, the community burden of *Plasmodium* parasite, and mortality associated with malaria.[8] Because there are no known risks associated with the use of insecticide-treated bed nets, usage should be encouraged in any prospective traveler to a malaria endemic area.

Other basic counseling should stress the need for general protection against insect bites. This has additive benefit, because preventative solutions that reduce mosquito bites also protect against most insect-borne disease (eg, ones not prevented by bed nets or malaria chemoprophylaxis, such as dengue and rickettsial disease). Long sleeves and pants should be encouraged (which also afford protection from sunburn). If possible, permethrin impregnation should also be used, because this has been demonstrated to both reduce insect bites through clothing by 99% and insect bites of unprotected persons in the nearby area by 94%.[9] All of the bites in subjects wearing permethrin-coated clothes were in areas of uncovered skin. Therefore, use of oil-based repellents, such as picaridin or diethyltoluamide (DEET), should be encouraged in conjunction with protective clothing. DEET concentrations should be at least 24%, because lower concentrations are less reliably effective.[10]

Step 3: Prescribe Chemoprophylaxis

Preventative medications (chemoprophylaxis) should be offered to any person traveling to an area where malaria is prevalent (**Table 1**). When taken properly, they are highly effective in preventing malaria acquisition. For example, in a Dutch study, none of 653 patients who took appropriate prophylaxis was diagnosed with clinical malaria.[11] The degree of protection, however, probably depends on exposure. In studies of US military personnel in Somalia, breakthrough infections were described in patients with documented therapeutic levels of both doxycycline and mefloquine.[12] In the Somali experience, guard duty near the Jubba River, where bite intensity was high, was identified as a strong risk factor.

Noncompliance is a major obstacle to effective chemoprophylaxis and has been repeatedly identified as a risk factor for development of clinical malaria. Typically, chemoprophylaxis is intended for persons with a time-limited exposure to malaria, when sustainable compliance is realistic. The early parasite stages are resistant to medication effect, so all agents must be continued for some period of time after exposure, from 1 to 4 weeks depending on the drug, which further complicates adherence.

The role of long-term chemoprophylaxis for persons living in an endemic area needs to be discussed on an individual basis. Studies of compliance in long-term expatriates have demonstrated that willingness to take long-term prophylaxis drops dramatically (to <40% of the population) beyond approximately 3 months recommended therapy.[13]

There are several options for chemoprophylaxis and no head-to-head superiority trials exist. All Food and Drug Administration–approved regimens have been highly effective—when patients are compliant—and well tolerated.[11] Therefore, the choice of drug can be customized based on patient preference, side-effect profile, and cost. In large surveys of European travelers, atovaquone/proguanil is the most frequently prescribed agent for short-term travelers (defined as less than 3 months) whereas mefloquine is generally recommended for long-term travel.

Geographic considerations: new world versus old world

Leading options for chemoprophylaxis include doxycycline, mefloquine, and atovaquone/proguanil. Although antifolate drugs (trimethoprim/sulfamethoxazole and sulfadoxine/pyrimethamine) are active against malaria, the parasite has developed resistance to these agents in sub-Saharan Africa, and they have failed in clinical trials of prophylaxis in pregnant women.

Chloroquine Although previously a mainstay of malaria treatment, this agent cannot be used outside of limited situations. At this time, the only areas with reliably susceptible *Plasmodium* parasites are in Latin America west of the Panama Canal (the Darién region has well described chloroquine resistant strains) and the Caribbean. Long-term use is associated with retinal toxicity and the agent is contraindicated in patients with a history of psoriasis or epilepsy. In general, it is well tolerated, as evidenced by the safe long-term use of its derivative (hydroxychloroquine) in patients with systemic lupus erythematosus. A long half-life allows for once-weekly dosing. It is safe in pregnancy.

Advantages: safe, well tolerated, usually affordable
Drawbacks: worldwide resistance outside Caribbean
Target population: potential travelers to Caribbean (eg, Haiti)
Typical adult dose: 500 mg salt (300 mg base) by mouth weekly, starting 2 weeks pre-exposure and continuing for 4 weeks postexposure

Table 1
Malaria chemoprophylaxis summary

Drug	Reasons to Consider Using This Drug	Reasons to Consider Avoiding This Drug
Atovaquone/ proguanil (Malarone)	• Good for last-minute travelers because the drug is started 1–2 d before traveling to an area where malaria transmission occurs • Some patients prefer to take a daily medicine. • Good choice for shorter trips because it is only taken for 7 d after traveling rather than 4 wk • Very well tolerated—side effects uncommon • Pediatric tablets are available and may be more convenient	• Cannot be used by women who are pregnant or breastfeeding a child <5 kg • Cannot be taken by people with severe renal impairment • Tends to be more expensive than some of the other options (especially for trips of long duration) • Some patients (including children) would rather not take a dose every day.
Chloroquine	• Some people would rather take medicine weekly. • Good choice for long trips because it is taken only weekly • Some people are already taking hydroxychloroquine chronically for rheumatologic conditions. In those instances, they may not have to take an additional medicine. • Can be used in all trimesters of pregnancy	• Cannot be used in areas with chloroquine or mefloquine resistance • May exacerbate psoriasis • Some patients would rather not take a weekly medication. • For trips of short duration, some people would rather not take medication for 4 wk after travel. • Not a good choice for last-minute travelers because drug needs to be started 1–2 wk prior to travel
Doxycycline	• Some people prefer to take a daily medicine. • Good for last-minute travelers because the drug is started 1–2 d before traveling to an area where malaria transmission occurs • Tends to be the least expensive antimalarial • Some people are already taking doxycycline chronically for prevention of acne. In those instances, they do not have to take an additional medicine. • Doxycycline also can prevent some additional infections (eg, rickettsiae and leptospirosis), so it may be preferred by people planning to do lots of hiking, camping, and wading and swimming in fresh water.	• Cannot be used by pregnant women and children <8 y old • Some people would rather not take a medicine every day • For trips of short duration, some people would rather not take medication for 4 wk after travel. • Women prone to getting vaginal yeast infections when taking antibiotics may prefer taking a different medicine. • Persons planning on considerable sun exposure may want to avoid the increased risk of sun sensitivity. • Some people are concerned about the potential of getting an upset stomach from doxycycline.

(*continued on next page*)

Table 1
(*continued*)

Drug	Reasons to Consider Using This Drug	Reasons to Consider Avoiding This Drug
Mefloquine (Lariam)	• Some patients would rather take medicine weekly. • Good choice for long trips because it is taken only weekly • Can be used during pregnancy	• Cannot be used in areas with mefloquine resistance • Cannot be used in patients with certain psychiatric conditions • Cannot be used in patients with a seizure disorder • Not recommended for persons with cardiac conduction abnormalities • Not a good choice for last-minute travelers because drug needs to be started at least 2 wk prior to travel • Some patients would rather not take a weekly medication. • For trips of short duration, some people would rather not take medication for 4 wk after travel.

From Centers for Disease Control and Prevention. Choosing a drug to prevent malaria. Available at: http://www.cdc.gov/malaria/travelers/drugs.html. Accessed August 26, 2015.

Mefloquine Mefloquine is active against chloroquine-resistant strains and has a prolonged half-life that allows for once-weekly dosing and may mitigate the consequences of a slightly delayed dose. This makes it an attractive agent for persons who are going to be in malarious areas for a prolonged period of time. In studies of 369 US military personnel deployed to Somalia, mefloquine was better tolerated than doxycycline, with skin photosensitivity and gastrointestinal symptoms occurring in 20% to 30% of patients taking doxycycline versus 5% to 10% of patients taking mefloquine. No differences were observed in the rates of neuropsychiatric effects.

There is some controversy with respect to the neuropsychiatric effects of mefloquine. There are well-described adverse events, including severe neuropsychiatric incidents, and the medication carries a warning label for patients with a history of psychiatric disorder. In general, the rate of neuropsychiatric problems is higher in women than with comparator drugs. The major symptoms were headache and sleep disturbances.[11] The authors' opinion is that the risk of neuropsychiatric effects is in general overstated and that the rate of adverse reactions is low in both clinical practice and epidemiologic studies. Still, the risks and benefits should be discussed with prospective patients. Special caution should be applied to situations wherein patients cannot seek medical attention or are in a remote or isolated situation.

Mefloquine is metabolized in the liver by cytochrome P450 3A4. Hepatic metabolism leads to many potential drug interactions, which should be considered prior to prescription of mefloquine. It is safe in pregnancy.

Advantages: once-weekly dosing makes ideal long-term regimen; little resistance
Drawbacks: minority of patients experience neuropsychiatric effects; many drug interactions (cytochrome P450 3A4)
Target: Peace Corps volunteers in remote areas; long-term volunteers or employees

Typical adult dose: 250 mg salt (228 mg base) by mouth weekly, starting 2 to 3 weeks pre-exposure and continuing 4 weeks postexposure

Atovaquone/proguanil Atovaquone/proguanil is a coformulated drug that acts synergistically against the malaria parasite and can be used for either treatment or prophylaxis. Atovaquone itself was found inadequate as monotherapy for treatment of established malaria infections and rapidly induces resistance, so the authors do not recommend use as monotherapy.

One particular advantage of atovaquone/proguanil is that it has activity against the liver stage. Therefore, patients do not have to take the medication for as long as other prophylactic options on return from a malarious area. The Food and Drug Administration package insert recommends taking the medication for 1 week on return from a malarious area, and the authors support this practice. In Israel, however, a frequent recommendation is to cease taking the medication 1 day after return. Passive surveillance has detected no failures with the 1 day after return from an endemic area duration of chemoprophylaxis.[14] It is probably safe during gestation, but conclusive trials are lacking, thus its official status: contraindicated in pregnancy.

Advantages: effective, well tolerated; only need to take for short course on return
Disadvantages: expensive
Target: short-term exposure to malarious area
Typical adult dose: 250 mg atovaquone + 100 mg proguanil by mouth daily, starting 2 days pre-exposure and continuing for 7 days postexposure

Doxycycline Doxycycline can be used as monotherapy for prophylaxis of malaria but not for treatment. Like all malaria chemoprophylaxis agents, it is in general well tolerated. There are 2 specific risks highlighted. The most common risk is esophageal irritation. In general, this is the most common side effect but can be mitigated with precautionary advice. In a population of Dutch patients, no esophageal irritation was determined. Patients were counseled to take the pill with a glass of water after food and not to take the pill at least 1 hour prior to lying supine.[11] Because this antibiotic is effective against leptospirosis and rickettsial infections, it may be advantageous for patients in whom there is a high likelihood of exposure to fresh water or tick bites. It is contraindicated in pregnancy.

Advantages: effective, well tolerated; has activity against other potential pathogens, including leptospirosis, rickettsia
Disadvantages: esophageal irritation/ulceration; skin photosensitivity; price varies unpredictably
Target: longer-term exposure in patients likely to use sun protection and/or be exposed to other zoonotic pathogens (eg, safari)
Typical adult dose: 100 mg by mouth daily starting 2 days pre-exposure and continuing 4 weeks postexposure

Step 4: Educate on Warning Signs of Malaria

For travelers going to an area where malaria is endemic, predeparture counseling is an important element of malaria prevention. Advice has been shown to reduce the risk of both insect bites and malaria acquisition.[15] Most patients have heard of malaria but have little understanding of what causes it, how it presents, or what the consequences may be. This can lead to both poor prevention compliance and delayed presentation to medical attention if clinical malaria develops—which can have life-threatening consequences. Patients who are returning to an area from which they immigrated are also at risk, because naturally acquired immunity wanes after leaving an endemic area. They should be offered advice and chemoprophylaxis the same as persons who have never been to an endemic area. A majority of patients diagnosed with malaria in 2012 in the United States (66%) were returning from visiting friends and relatives, with more than 90% returning from sub-Saharan Africa.[2]

All patients should be referred to www.CDC.gov/malaria, which has excellent teaching materials. They should also be told these fundamental facts:

- Careful prevention techniques (bite avoidance and chemoprophylaxis) are excellent but not perfect.
- Fever may be malaria, up to a year after coming home from an endemic area.
- Malaria can turn dangerous quickly, and early diagnosis and treatment can save your life. Any fever should trigger a call or visit to a medical doctor for prompt assessment, up to a year after returning. Tell your health care provider that you were exposed to malaria.
- Even if you have lived in an endemic area for a long time, and even if you have had malaria before, you can get it again, and it can be serious every time.

CLINICAL PRESENTATION: ALWAYS SUSPECT MALARIA IN AN ILL RETURNING TRAVELER

Take-home points

- Flulike symptoms are most common presentation.
- Clinical presentation of malaria is nonspecific.
- Cyclic fevers are not characteristic of malaria.
- Diarrhea and abdominal pain are common.
- Malaria may copresent with other sources of fever.

Malaria should be suspected in any patient with a febrile syndrome after returning from a malarious area. The typical syndrome described for acute uncomplicated malaria is described as an influenza-like illness, with fever, myalgias, and headaches. An underappreciated element of the syndrome is gastrointestinal illness. The pathophysiologic explanation for why patients who are immunologically naive experience abdominal pain and diarrhea is unclear, and this presentation differs from patients who experience malaria in an endemic area. But the bottom line is that acute malaria often presents with diarrhea.

The classic tertian (every 48 hours) or quartian (every 72 hours) fever can still be found in many textbooks, but this pattern is rare among travelers, because it generally takes some time for the parasites to synchronize their life cycles. Clinicians should not consider the fever pattern in evaluating patients for malaria and have an extremely low threshold for further diagnostic testing. Malaria is a well-described cause of sepsis, and delays in treatment have been implicated in poor outcomes.[1]

Because there is a lag between the initial bite by an infected mosquito to progression and amplification in the liver stages of a parasite's life cycle, and eventually the development of symptomatic blood-stage infection, patients should be counseled (and providers should be aware) that clinical malaria can develop up to 1 year after return from a malaria endemic area. For a majority of patients, however, the incubation period is approximately 7 to 14 days. One hospital reported that the mean time of patients return from an endemic area and presentation to the hospital was 9.5 days (3–14).[16]

There are major differences in the life cycle between the 4 species of *Plasmodium* that infect humans and this difference should be explained to patients. *P falciparum*, the most common cause of malaria in travelers, is not associated with a residual liver stage. Therefore, if a patient is effectively treated and recovers, the chance of late relapse is extremely low. This is not the case for *P vivax* and *P ovale*, which have residual liver stages called *hypnozoites*. Therefore, even with adequate acute treatment a patient can experience relapse months or years later. Experiences with military veterans returning from the Korea war documented relapses up to 30 years after return (with no subsequent exposure). In more recent studies of Australian military personnel who were treated for malaria with *P vivax* infections during deployment to East Timor, relapses happened approximately 9 months after a clinical infection (median 180 days).[17] The longest documented relapse was 777 days.

Finally, malaria should remain on the differential diagnosis and ruled out definitively even if an alternative source of fever is detected in a returning traveler. Respiratory infections, gastrointestinal infections, or urinary infections may coexist with malaria, and should not distract a provider from continuing to rule out malaria, especially when patients fail to respond to treatment.

DIAGNOSIS

Take-home points

- Thick and thin smears are useful for prognosis but are operator dependent.
- Rapid diagnostic tests can be quickly used to distinguish *Babesia* from malaria.

Smear

Despite being used for over a century,[18] microscopic evaluation of peripheral blood smear remains the only technique for which qualitative, quantitative, and prognostic factors are assessed in 1 inexpensive test. The reagents for preparing a peripheral smear should be available at most large health care facilities: Wright-Giemsa stain, slides, and a microscope. Unfortunately, the human element of technologists and clinicians familiar with malaria varies considerably between institutions. In general, areas of lower prevalence and less experience with malaria have less reliable smear microscopic evaluation.

Smears are always ordered in pairs: thick and thin. The thick smear is approximately 30 times as sensitive as the thin smear, because much more blood is used on each slide; however, thick smears do not provide reliable information on the species or burden of infection. Thin smears show the parasites clearly and allow a skillful operator to identify the species and count the parasitemia at the same time.

A single negative pair of smears does not exclude a diagnosis of malaria. This is because of the episodic nature of parasitemia, in which detectable parasites may appear on the smear at 1 point in the day, then disappear hours later. Thus, ideally, smears should be repeated every 8 hours for 48 hours to achieve an optimal negative predictive value. The Thai experience is illustrative, because the clinical laboratories in Thailand are thought to have some of the highest-quality microscopists. When experienced microscopists were asked to evaluate smears, the diagnostic yield had a false-negative rate of approximately 10% to 15% compared with more stringent research analysis conducted as part of the Armed Forces Research Institute of Medical Sciences.[18] Furthermore, clinicians should be aware that false-positive results are also possible (in the Thai experience, these were more common than false-negative results, at approximately 25%). The rates of both false-positive results and false-negative results were strongly influenced by the density of parasites in the blood, because lower densities of parasites were strongly associated with both false-positive results and false negative results. Caution should be advised because platelets, red blood cell fragments, and staining artifacts are all reported to be confused with malaria parasites. Malaria co-infection can also occur, so even with a firm diagnosis of malaria, clinicians should seek to exclude alternative explanations for febrile syndromes if the patient does not respond to antimalarial therapies.

Rapid Diagnostic Tests

Rapid diagnostics are based on the same immunochromatographic technology as standard home pregnancy test (**Fig. 2**). Most rapid diagnostics use blood from finger pricks (although venous blood works). In general, rapid diagnostics offer comparable sensitivity to smear microscopy with much less interobserver variability. There are a variety of different brands, but in general the target of the bands is a malarial antigen expressed in blood-stage infection. Some brands differentiate between the various malaria species, whereas others do not. It is important for clinicians to be aware of the difference in brands. Health care providers in nonendemic areas often underuse these valuable tests, although the use of rapid diagnostics has been demonstrated safe in a nonendemic population.[19]

Furthermore, the antigen-specific nature of the rapid diagnostic testing can be useful in areas where both *Babesia* species are endemic and/or babesiosis is suspected based on epidemiologic exposure (eg, in the setting of a tick bite in a recently returned traveler). There is no antigenic cross-reactivity between the malaria antigens used in rapid diagnostic testing and *Babesia spp.*; therefore, a patient with intraerythrocytic parasites on smear who has a negative rapid diagnostic test is likely to have *Babesiosis*.

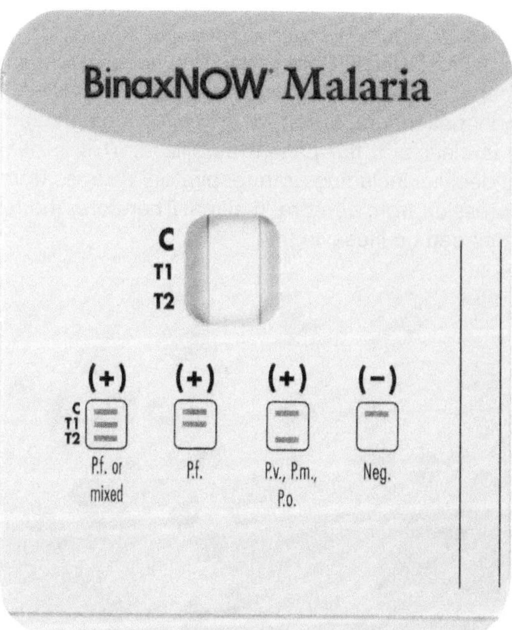

Fig. 2. Rapid diagnostic test for malaria. Some training is required to perform and interpret this assay but much less than for blood smears. (© 2015 Alere. All rights reserved. BinaxNOW is a trademark of the Alere group of companies. Photo permission granted by Alere.)

Species Difference: Clinical Considerations

For the generalist, the largest distinction in smear microscopy should be made between infections with *P falciparum* and nonfalciparum species. *P falciparum* is responsible for a majority of imported disease, is associated with more severe disease (discussed later), and requires treatment different from the other species. Furthermore, occasionally other blood-borne parasites are observed and smear microscopy should be considered to look for other types of blood-stage parasitic infections in the febrile patient returning from an area where malaria is endemic. Even in centers with ready access to rapid molecular diagnostics, the authors recommend that all patients with suspected or confirmed malaria receive a peripheral smear.

Caution should be advised, because mixed infections can happen in most areas of the world. Even in areas with experienced microscopists, 10% of patients diagnosed with *P vivax* infections (associated with less severe disease) actually have *P falciparum* compared with the reference standard of polymerase chain reaction–based species identification.[20] In general, *P falciparum* typically has mostly ring stages in peripheral smear (**Fig. 3**).

TREATMENT

- Seek expert opinion.
- Consider inpatient admission and treat as sepsis syndrome.
- Artemisinin-based compounds are standard of care but not always readily available.
- For severe infection, initiate treatment with quinidine while awaiting further guidance.

Treatment of malaria is beyond the scope of this article. For clinicians unfamiliar with malaria, the authors advise seeking expert advice immediately on making a diagnosis of malaria. The Centers for Disease Control and Prevention maintains an active hotline with excellent clinical advice available 24 hours a day: 770-488-7100. In general, the authors recommend inpatient admission for any patient diagnosed with malaria until the clinical course is clear and the patient stabilized. This is because malaria can cause rapid clinical decline, including both respiratory distress from acute lung injury and respiratory depression from cerebral malaria. Therefore, the ready availability of critical care resources can be lifesaving.

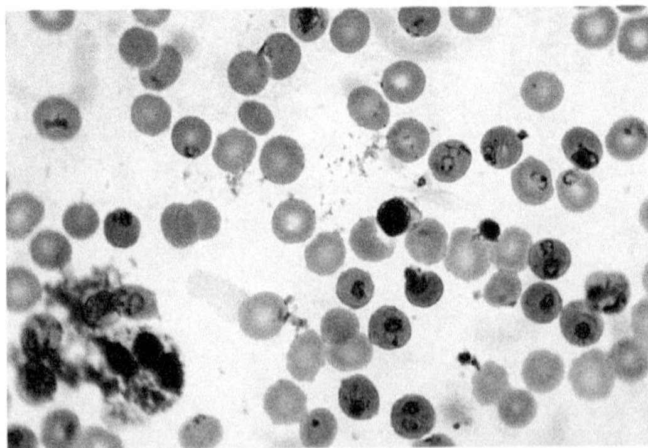

Fig. 3. Thin smear of *P falciparum* malaria. Note high burden of parasites, which look like signet rings or headphones within multiply infected normal-sized erythrocytes, all hallmarks of *P falciparum* (Wright-Giemsa stain, original magnification x100).

Although nonfalciparum malaria is generally treatable with chloroquine, the consequences of treating drug-resistant falciparum malaria this way can be grave. Thus, if there is any doubt whatsoever regarding the species involved, treat presumptively for falciparum.

In general, artemisinin-based compounds are recommended as standard of care for falciparum malaria. This is because these drugs rapidly kill all stages of the parasite, and clinical trials in endemic populations have demonstrated mortality benefit compared with intravenous quinine. The problem is that these compounds may not be readily available at all centers. Uncomplicated malaria can be treated with oral artemether/lumefantrine, atovaquone/proguanil, or quinine plus doxycycline, whereas complicated or severe malaria should be treated in an ICU with parenteral artesunate, quinidine plus clindamycin, or doxycycline. Time is of the essence in treating malaria and, therefore, the authors recommend initiating treatment immediately with any effective antifalciparum compound available while seeking expert consultation. In the authors' experience, parenteral quinidine is more commonly available because of its utility as an antiarrhythmic.

REFERENCES

1. Harvey K, Esposito DH, Han P, et al. Surveillance for travel-related disease–GeoSentinel Surveillance System, United States, 1997-2011. MMWR Surveill Summ 2013;62:1–23.
2. Cullen KA, Arguin PM, Centers for Disease Control and Prevention (CDC). Malaria surveillance–United States, 2012. MMWR Surveill Summ 2014;63:1–22.
3. Elliott JH, O'Brien D, Leder K, et al. Imported Plasmodium vivax malaria: demographic and clinical features in nonimmune travelers. J Travel Med 2004;11: 213–7.
4. Siala E, Gamara D, Kallel K, et al. Airport malaria: report of four cases in Tunisia. Malar J 2015;14:42.
5. Whitworth J, Morgan D, Quigley M, et al. Effect of HIV-1 and increasing immunosuppression on malaria parasitaemia and clinical episodes in adults in rural Uganda: a cohort study. Lancet 2000;356:1051–6.
6. Bach O, Baier M, Pullwitt A, et al. Falciparum malaria after splenectomy: a prospective controlled study of 33 previously splenectomized Malawian adults. Trans R Soc Trop Med Hyg 2005;99:861–7.
7. Oster CN, Koontz LC, Wyler DJ. Malaria in asplenic mice: effects of splenectomy, congenital asplenia, and splenic reconstitution on the course of infection. Am J Trop Med Hyg 1980;29:1138–42.
8. Lengeler C. Insecticide-treated bed nets and curtains for preventing malaria Cochrane Database of Systematic Reviews 2004, Issue 2. Art. No.: CD000363.
9. Schreck CE, Haile DG, Kline DL. The effectiveness of permethrin and deet, alone or in combination, for protection against Aedes taeniorhynchus. Am J Trop Med Hyg 1984;33:725–30.
10. Fradin MS, Day JF. Comparative efficacy of insect repellents against mosquito bites. N Engl J Med 2002;347:13–8.
11. Schlagenhauf P, Tschopp A, Johnson R, et al. Tolerability of malaria chemoprophylaxis in non-immune travellers to sub-Saharan Africa: multicentre, randomised, double blind, four arm study. BMJ 2003;327:1078.
12. Wallace MR, Sharp TW, Smoak B, et al. Malaria among United States troops in Somalia. Am J Med 1996;100:49–55.

13. Cunningham J, Horsley J, Patel D, et al. Compliance with long-term malaria prophylaxis in British expatriates. Travel Med Infect Dis 2014;12:341–8.
14. Leshem E, Meltzer E, Stienlauf S, et al. Effectiveness of short prophylactic course of atovaquone-proguanil in travelers to sub-saharan Africa. J Trav Med 2014;21:82–5.
15. Tafuri S, Guerra R, Gallone MS, et al. Effectiveness of pre-travel consultation in the prevention of travel-related diseases: a retrospective cohort study. Trav Med Infect Dis 2014;12:745–9.
16. Marks ME, Armstrong M, Suvari MM, et al. Severe imported falciparum malaria among adults requiring intensive care: a retrospective study at the hospital for tropical diseases, London. BMC Infect Dis 2013;13:118.
17. Chen N, Auliff A, Rieckmann K, et al. Relapses of Plasmodium vivax infection result from clonal hypnozoites activated at predetermined intervals. J Infect Dis 2007;195:934–41.
18. McKenzie FE, Sirichaisinthop J, Miller RS, et al. Dependence of malaria detection and species diagnosis by microscopy on parasite density. Am J Trop Med Hyg 2003;69:372–6.
19. Rossi IA, D'Acremont V, Prod'Hom G, et al. Safety of falciparum malaria diagnostic strategy based on rapid diagnostic tests in returning travellers and migrants: a retrospective study. Malar J 2012;11:377.
20. Mekonnen SK, Aseffa A, Medhin G, et al. Re-evaluation of microscopy confirmed Plasmodium falciparum and Plasmodium vivax malaria by nested PCR detection in southern Ethiopia. Malar J 2014;13:48.

Personal Protection Measures Against Mosquitoes, Ticks, and Other Arthropods

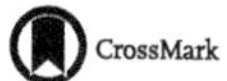

Jonathan D. Alpern, MD[a,*], Stephen J. Dunlop, MD, MPH, CTropMed[b], Benjamin J. Dolan, MD[c], William M. Stauffer, MD, MSPH[d], David R. Boulware, MD, MPH, CTropMed[e]

KEYWORDS

• Arthropod bites • Personal protection measures • Travelers • Mosquitoes
• Repellants • DEET • Ticks

KEY POINTS

- Bite avoidance and personal protection measures should be recommended to all travelers.
- Traveler characteristics and destination-specific factors should be considered when deciding which personal protection measures to recommend.
- DEET, picaridin, PMD, and IR3535 are insect repellents that provide adequate protection for travelers against arthropod bites, with the exception of IR3535, which should not be recommended for use in malaria-endemic areas.
- Insecticide-treated clothing in combination with topical insect repellents provides nearly complete protection against arthropod bites.
- In addition to repellents, further methods of modifying the environment, such as insecticide-treated bed nets should be recommended, particularly for travelers to malaria-endemic areas.

Disclosure Statement: The authors have no disclosures or conflicts of interest.

[a] Division of Infectious Disease & International Medicine, University of Minnesota, 420 Delaware Street SE, MMC 250 Mayo, Minneapolis, MN 55455, USA; [b] Department of Emergency Medicine, Hennepin County Medical Center, University of Minnesota, 701 Park Avenue, Minneapolis, MN 55415, USA; [c] Department of Emergency Medicine, Hennepin County Medical Center, 701 Park Avenue, Minneapolis, MN 55415, USA; [d] Division of Infectious Diseases & International Medicine, Department of Medicine, University of Minnesota, 420 Delaware Street Southeast, 133 Variety Club Research Center, MMC 284, Minneapolis, MN 55455, USA; [e] Infectious Disease & International Medicine, Department of Medicine, University of Minnesota, MTRF 3-222, 2001 6th Street Southeast, Minneapolis, MN 55455, USA
* Corresponding author.
E-mail address: alper054@umn.edu

Med Clin N Am 100 (2016) 303–316
http://dx.doi.org/10.1016/j.mcna.2015.08.019 medical.theclinics.com

INTRODUCTION

Arthropod-associated diseases are a major cause of morbidity in travelers. Arthropods are defined as invertebrate animals with an exoskeleton, segmented body, and jointed appendages, and include mosquitoes, ticks, flies, and chiggers. Among ill returning travelers presenting to travel and tropical medicine clinics, vector-borne diseases (malaria, dengue, and rickettsia) accounted for most systemic febrile illnesses.[1] In another study, malaria and dengue were the most common causes of illness among travelers returning from Sub-Saharan Africa, Latin America, Caribbean, Southeast Asia, Australia, New Zealand, and Oceana.[2] The recent emergence of the chikungunya virus into the Western hemisphere reinforces the importance of mosquito bite avoidance and other personal protective measures as the primary means of protecting travelers from vector-borne diseases.[3,4] Despite being effective, compliance with personal protection measures among travelers to malaria-endemic regions is poor.[5] The pretravel visit serves an important role for vector-borne disease prevention that should not be overlooked. Pretravel advice was associated with a reduced risk of malaria, and malaria-associated morbidity across traveler groups.[6] This article reviews the personal protection measures available for travelers, the evidence behind them, and recommendations for their use in the prevention of arthropod bites in travelers (**Fig. 1**).

DESTINATION AND VECTOR CONSIDERATIONS

During the pretravel visit, obtaining a detailed travel itinerary is a key aspect of risk assessment. The planned destination, urban versus rural setting, length of stay, modes of transportation, reason for visit, and accommodation all affect one's risk for arthropod exposures and subsequent vector-borne diseases. Having an understanding of the arthropod vectors present at one's destination is essential to adequately advising the traveler on mitigating risk. For instance, the *Anopheles* mosquito, which transmits malaria, is primarily a nighttime-biting arthropod, and insecticide-treated bed nets may augment repellents and other measures taken, such as chemoprophylactic drugs, when traveling to malaria-endemic areas. Conversely, dengue and chikungunya are viral diseases transmitted by the daytime-biting *Aedes* mosquitoes. Therefore, insect repellents and protective clothing should

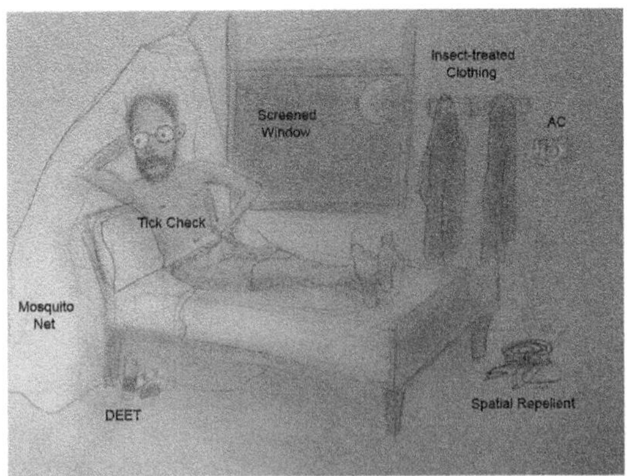

Fig. 1. "Chance favors only the prepared mind" - Louis Pasteur. Traveler with personal protection measures. (*Courtesy of* Benjamin J. Dolan, MD, Hennepin County Medical Center.)

be stressed for travelers visiting endemic regions. The characteristics of other common medically important arthropods relevant to travelers and the associated diseases they transmit can be seen in **Table 1**.

TRAVELER CONSIDERATIONS

In addition to considering destination-specific risk factors, individual traveler-specific characteristics also should be considered when assessing risk. Some types of travelers are at greater risk of vector-borne disease than others. Higher-risk travelers may be stratified based on age, purpose of their trip, and activities during the trip. Younger age is a risk factor for nonadherence to health prevention measures during travel.[7,8] "Visiting Friends and Relatives" (VFR) travelers, defined as travelers who visit friends or relatives in locations that create a gradient of health risk (both infectious and noninfectious) when compared with the departure country,[9] are at increased risk of travel-related health problems, including malaria.[10] This is likely due to multiple factors, including higher-risk destinations, longer stays, less pre-travel advice, decreased use of protective measures, and a false sense of immunity.[11] Further stratifying VFRs into "immigrant VFR" and "traveler VFR" (ie, second-generation immigrants or children of immigrant VFRs) reveals a heterogeneous population with regard to travel-related health risk. Immigrant VFRs are at greater risk of acquiring malaria, and of those becoming ill were less likely to have sought pretravel advice when compared with the traveler VFR and non-VFR tourist travelers.[10]

Adventure travelers also may be at increased risk of arthropod bites and vector-borne diseases. Adventure travel is an increasingly popular form of tourism that combines physical activity, a connection to the environment, and cultural immersion.[12] Adventure travel and backpacking were the most common forms of travel in patients presenting with a skin disorder to travel and tropical medicine clinics.[13] An outbreak of African tick bite fever (*Rickettsia africae*; transmitted by ticks) occurred in 13 French adventure racers in rural South Africa.[14] Adventure travelers who spend time in forests in the evening are at high risk of cutaneous leishmaniasis (*Leishmania* protozoa; transmitted by the sand fly).[15] Other activities may also predispose to vector-borne diseases, including hiking and camping (eg, tick-borne encephalitis in Europe),[16] hunting (eg, African tick-bite fever in South Africa),[17] and safari (eg, trypanosomiasis in Tanzania and Kenya).[18]

General Protective Measures

- *Avoidance:* Travelers should avoid areas with known outbreaks and epidemics, and be aware of peak exposure times and places. Heavily vegetated areas, which are often inhabited by ticks and chiggers, should be avoided if possible.[19] The use of air conditioning was associated with a reduced incidence of malaria among travelers to a malaria-endemic area.[5] When in malaria-endemic areas, being in a protected environment during the evening and nighttime hours may reduce risk of exposure (eg, well-screened dwellings, air-conditioned rooms, using a fan).
- *Bed nets:* Especially if rooms are not screened or air conditioned, bed nets offer protection against nighttime-biting arthropod vectors and nuisance biting. Bed nets are most effective when treated with a pyrethroid insecticide (ie, permethrin)[20] either before or during travel.
- *Spatial repellents:* Devices that repel mosquitoes from a distance have gained in popularity, and include impregnated plastic strips, coils, candles, fan emanators, and heat-generating devices.[21] Spatial repellents can be used to clear the

Table 1
Arthropods relevant to travelers and recommendations for personal protection measures

Disease	Pathogen	Arthropod Vector	Biting Times	Greatest Risk of Transmission	Location	Most Important Personal Protection Method
Malaria	*Plasmodium* protozoa	*Anopheles* mosquito	Dusk to dawn	• During/following the rainy season[20]	Africa, Latin America, parts of the Caribbean, Asia, Eastern Europe, and South Pacific	• Nighttime mosquito avoidance: topical insect repellents, protective clothing, well-screened or air-conditioned rooms, insecticide-treated bed net (ITN), and insecticide aerosol sprays in sleeping areas • Chemoprophylaxis
Dengue	Dengue virus	*Aedes aegypti* and *Aedes albopictus* mosquitoes	Daytime	• Following rainy season and during epidemics[20]	Central and South America, Caribbean, Africa, Middle East, Asia, Oceana	• Daytime mosquito avoidance: insect repellents, personal protective clothing, insecticide-treated clothing • Empty nearby containers that have standing water
Chikungunya	Chikungunya virus	*Aedes aegypti* and *Aedes albopictus* mosquitoes	Daytime	• During epidemics, tropical rainy season • Can also occur during dry season when there is abundant standing water	Africa, Asia, Europe, South America, Central America, Islands on the Pacific and Indian Ocean	• Daytime mosquito avoidance: insect repellents, personal protective clothing, insecticide-treated clothing • Empty nearby containers that have standing water

West Nile virus	West Nile virus	*Culex* mosquito	Dusk and dawn	• Year round in tropics, warmer months in northern hemisphere[20]	North America, Europe, Central and South America, Caribbean, Africa, Middle East, Australia[43]	• Mosquito avoidance: topical insect repellents, protective clothing, well-screened or air-conditioned rooms, ITN, and insecticide aerosol sprays in sleeping areas
Yellow fever	Yellow fever virus	*Aedes aegypti* mosquitoes	Daytime	• West Africa: End of rainy season, beginning of dry season (ie, July–October). Occasionally during dry season • South America: Rainy season (January – May)[44]	Africa, South and Central America[44]	• Vaccination • Mosquito bite avoidance
Japanese encephalitis	Japanese encephalitis virus	*Culex* mosquito	Dusk and dawn	• Primarily in rural agricultural areas • In temperate areas of Asia: transmission peaks in summer/fall. • In tropics/subtropics: varies with monsoon rains; may occur year-round[45]	Asia and Western Pacific[45]	• Vaccination • Mosquito bite avoidance
Leishmaniasis	*Leishmania* protozoa	Sand fly	Dusk to dawn, or during the day if disturbed in habitat[46]	• Year round	Every continent except Australia and Antarctica[47]	• Sand fly avoidance: avoid outdoor activities especially at night, protective clothing, insect repellent, insecticide-treated clothing, use well-screened or air-conditioned rooms • ITN: smaller mesh size needed[46]

(*continued on next page*)

Table 1
(*continued*)

Disease	Pathogen	Arthropod Vector	Biting Times	Greatest Risk of Transmission	Location	Most Important Personal Protection Method
Scrub typhus	*Orientia tsutsugamushi*	Larval mites (chigger)	Day and night	• Visits to rural areas in endemic countries	Northern Japan, Southeast Asia, western Pacific islands, Eastern Australia, China, south central Russia, India, and Sri Lanka[48]	• Minimize exposure when traveling in endemic areas. • Avoidance measures: insect repellents, protective clothing, insecticide-treated clothing
African tick-bite fever	*Rickettsia africae*	Ticks	Day and night	• Game hunting, and travel to southern Africa during the months of November – April[48]	Sub-Saharan Africa, West Indies	• Minimize exposure when traveling in endemic areas. • Avoidance measures: insect repellents, protective clothing, insecticide-treated clothing • Check body after being in high-risk areas

bedroom of mosquitoes before sleeping, and coils and emanators do decrease the amount of contact between humans and mosquitoes.[22] However, data are limited on their effectiveness at preventing vector-borne diseases, and should be used only in addition to other proven, personal protection measures.

- *Protective clothing:* Wearing long-sleeve, loose-fitting shirts and trousers when traveling to malaria and other endemic regions has been shown to reduce the incidence of malaria among travelers.[5] *Despite this, compliance remains low among some groups,*[7] perhaps due to lower perceived risk, as well as hot and humid environments that can make compliance difficult. Neutral-colored clothing should be worn, as mosquitoes,[23] *tsetse flies,*[24] *and sand flies*[25] *appear to be attracted to dark colors.*
- *Check for ticks:* Travelers should inspect their body and clothing for ticks immediately after outdoor activity and at the end of the day.

TOPICAL INSECT REPELLENTS

The active chemical ingredient, its concentration, and resultant duration of protection are the most important considerations when choosing an insect repellent.[26] The Centers for Disease Control and Prevention (CDC) has identified 4 active ingredients found in over-the-counter Environmental Protection Agency (EPA)-registered products with sufficient evidence for protection against arthropod bites in travelers.[19] A table summarizing the characteristics of the 4 insect repellents can be found in **Table 2**. In addition to considering the effectiveness of the product against destination-specific vectors, other factors that influence the product's effectiveness and duration of protection include the following:

- *Product formulation:* Multiple formulations are available; however, effectiveness varies depending on the product and arthropod species.
- *Concentration:* In general, the higher the concentration of the product, the greater the duration of protection.
- *Environmental conditions:* Rain, wind, and high temperatures can decrease a product's duration.
- *Biting density:* At a given time or place, the number of feeding arthropods may be higher than usual, and one should consider higher-concentration formulas and frequent reapplication in these circumstances.
- *User characteristics:* High activity level with associated increased evaporation and absorption, as well as wash-off sweat, may decrease the duration of protection. In addition, some individuals are more attractive to mosquitoes than others.[27]

TOPICAL INSECT REPELLENTS

N,N-diethyl-m-toluamide

N,N-diethyl-m-toluamide (DEET) is a broad-spectrum insect repellent, first developed by the US Department of Agriculture in 1946 for use by the US military.[28] Marketing for the product began in 1957, and it is now the most widely used and studied insect repellent available.[29] Products are sold in multiple formulations, including aerosols, pump sprays, lotions, creams, gels, towelettes, and wristbands. Products include Off! (SC Johnson, Racine, WI), Repel, Cutter (United Industries, Beloit, WI), Sawyer (Sawyer Products, Safety Harbor, FL), and Ultrathon (3M, St. Paul, MN). Although a consensus on its mechanism is lacking, multiple pathways modulating insect olfactory receptors are involved.[30] It is considered the gold standard insect repellent by the

Table 2
Summary of insect repellents

Agent	Protective Effect	Duration	Benefits	Limitations	Pregnancy and Breast Feeding	Safety	Age Range
DEET	DEET (20%–50%) protects against *Anopheles*, *Aedes*, and *Culex* mosquitoes	6–13 h	Most-studied insect repellent available	Foul smell and oily texture may limit use Can damage plastics	Safe in second and third trimester, and while breastfeeding Avoid in first trimester	Low risk of adverse events if used appropriately	>2 mo
Picaridin	Picaridin (20%) protects against *Anopheles*, *Aedes*, and *Culex* mosquitoes	5 h	Pleasant smell, less irritating to the skin than DEET Does not damage plastics	Shorter duration of action than DEET	Avoid	Safe for use, but limited data	>2 y[38]
PMD	PMD (30%) protects against *Anopheles*, *Aedes*, and *Culex* mosquitoes	4–6 h	Pleasant smell, less irritating to the skin than DEET Does not damage plastics	Shorter duration of action than DEET	Avoid	Safe for use but limited data	>3 y
IR3535	IR3535 (20%) protects against *Aedes* and *Culex* mosquitos, but does not adequately protect against *Anopheles*	7–10 h (*Aedes*, *Culex*) 3–4 h (*Anopheles*)	Nongreasy with no odor Does not damage plastics	Cannot be used in malaria-endemic areas	Avoid	Safe for use, with long history of use in Europe before US[49]	—

World Health Organization[31] and the CDC[32] for protection against malaria, and is the control by which other insect repellents are compared. Concentrations are available from 5% to 100%, with protection time proportional to concentration; a plateau effect occurs at approximately 50%. A concentration of 20% to 50% should be used in areas in which malaria and other vector-borne diseases are endemic, as this concentration has been shown to be the minimal amount needed to provide complete protection against *Aedes*, *Anopheles*, and *Culex* mosquitoes species for 6 to 13 hours.[26,33] The product should be reapplied every 6 to 8 hours for maximal protection.[26] Products with sustained or controlled-release formulations may provide longer protection times. For instance, an extended-duration formulation at 33% concentration showed adequate protection against ticks for 12 hours.[34] More studies are needed in this area, as previous studies have shown that DEET offers poor protection against ticks.[27]

Picaridin

Picaridin (KBR 3023), a derivative of piperidine, was first marketed in Europe in the 1990s and in the United States by 2005.[35] Products include Off!, Sawyer, and Skin So Soft Bug Guard Plus (Avon, New York, NY). The mechanism is unknown, although it is thought to involve a similar olfactory cofactor of DEET that discourages biting.[36] Picaridin 20% spray was shown to be comparable to 20% DEET for protection against *Aedes*, *Anopheles*, and *Culex* mosquito species, with no loss of protection over a 5-hour time period.[37] The product should be reapplied every 4 to 6 hours.[26] Unlike DEET, picaridin does not damage plastics and synthetics, and picaridin is less of a dermatologic and olfactory irritant.[38] Picaridin's comparable efficacy to DEET and favorable side-effect profile make it an appealing option and an acceptable alternative for protection against malaria and other vector-borne diseases in endemic areas.

p-Methane-3,8-diol (PMD) or Oil of Lemon Eucalyptus

PMD is derived from the oil of lemon-scented eucalyptus (OLE). Products include Repel (United Industries Corporation, Beloit, WI) and Cutter.[19] Of note, "pure" OLE has not been rigorously tested, is not registered by the EPA, and is not recommended for use here.[19] When used at concentrations of 30%, PMD offers complete protection for 4 to 6 hours against *Aedes*, *Anopheles*, and *Culex* spp,[26] and ticks.[33] It was shown to provide comparable protection against malaria as DEET and is recommended by the CDC for use in malaria-endemic areas. However, it has a shorter duration of protection than DEET, requiring more frequent application. In children, PMD should be used only in those older than 3 years.[26]

Ethyl Butylacetylaminopropionate (IR3535)

IR3535 is found in products including Skin So Soft Bug Guard Plus Expedition (Avon, New York, NY).[19] IR3535 20% offers complete protection against *Aedes* and *Culex* mosquitoes for 7 to 10 hours,[26] but only 3.8 hours of protection against *Anopheles* in some studies.[33] Therefore, IR3535 is not an adequate insect repellent option in malaria-endemic regions. The product should be reapplied every 6 to 8 hours.[26]

Safety

DEET safety

The risk of severe adverse events with DEET is low if used appropriately.[39] Although there has been controversy over the safety of DEET in children, DEET does appear safe for use in children older than 2 months.[26] Despite case reports of seizures and encephalopathy in children,[39] there are no data to suggest causation. According to the DEET Registry, risk of neurologic toxicity appears low, with no association between concentration and severity of disease.[28] DEET is also safe for use during the second and third trimesters of pregnancy with no adverse outcomes to the mother or fetus, based on a randomized double-blinded trial of pregnant women on the Thai-Burmese border.[40] Further studies are needed to evaluate its safety in the first trimester of pregnancy. DEET has been known to damage certain plastics (ie, glasses frames) and synthetic fabrics,[29] as well as spandex, rayon, acetate, and pigmented leather[38]; this effect is more likely in higher concentrations.

PMD, IR3535, and picaridin safety

The safety of DEET use in humans has been better studied than the other topical insect repellents. PMD, picaridin, and IR3535 are safe for use in nonpregnant individuals, but have not been studied during pregnancy and therefore should be avoided until further studies have been done.[26]

INSECTICIDE-TREATED CLOTHING, NETS, AND OTHER FABRICS

Permethrin

Permethrin is an odorless, biodegradable pyrethroid insecticide derived from the plant *Chrysanthemum cinerariifolium*. It is the most common insecticide available for use on fabrics, and is unique in its role as both a contact insecticide via neural toxicity, and as an insect repellent.[41] It requires direct contact with arthropods and is ineffective when applied directly to skin. It can be applied directly to clothing, as well as shoes, bed nets, and camping gear.[38]

Insecticide-Treated Clothing

Permethrin is the most common product used to treat clothing. Although intervention trials assessing the effect of insecticide-treated clothing on the risk of malaria, leishmaniasis, and scrub typhus have been mixed, when used in combination with topical insect repellents, insecticide-treated clothing offers close to 100% protection against arthropod bites.[41] It offers protection against mosquitoes, chigger mites, fleas, lice, sand flies, kissing bugs, and tsetse flies.[27] However the level of protection varies among mosquito species, with evidence for a high level of protection against *Anopheles* and *Aedes* spp, but low protection against *Culex* spp.[41] The method by which clothing is impregnated is important, and may affect efficacy, duration of protection, and cost. The absorption method involves dipping or spraying clothing with insecticide, and can be performed by the traveler or clothes can be pretreated. Individually treated clothing is more affordable, but offers less-consistent protection and does not last as long as pretreated clothing.[41] It is generally recommended that travelers who treat their clothing themselves reapply permethrin after 5 washes.[41] When applied appropriately, toxicity concerns are minimal.[20] The protection offered against a wide range of arthropod species, and minimal safety concerns, make permethrin-treated clothing an important arthropod-protection method when used in addition to other protection methods, including topical insect repellents.

Insecticide-Treated Bed Nets

Insecticide-treated bed nets (ITNs) are recommended for use in all travelers to malaria-endemic regions, as strong evidence exists for their effectiveness in the prevention of arthropod bites in travelers,[27] in addition to reducing indoor resting densities of malaria vectors in areas of high transmission.[42] However, ITNs need to be used regularly and retreated frequently to retain effectiveness.[42] Pyrethroid-treated nets last for several months if they are not washed.[19]

OTHER METHODS

Spatial Repellents and Aerosols

Insecticide vaporizers using permethrin prevent against nuisance biting but there is no evidence for prevention against malaria. In addition, travelers should be aware of a low-level health hazard risk and use these devices with caution.[27] Mosquito coils are effective against nuisance biting involving all mosquito species, and may reduce the risk of transmission of malaria. There have been concerns of an increased incidence of lung cancer in individuals using mosquito coils; however, given the minimal exposure expected for travelers, this appears to be a small risk.[27] Essential oil candles are another option for the prevention of nuisance biting, with some data suggesting effectiveness at bite prevention against mosquitoes and sandflies. However, there is no evidence for disease prevention. Finally, knockdown insecticide sprays, which are intended to be sprayed inside rooms, have not been shown to be effective at preventing malaria in travelers and may present a health risk due to the inhalation of vapors.[27]

FUTURE CONSIDERATIONS/SUMMARY

In conclusion, personal protection measures, which include protective clothing, topical insect repellents, and ITNs and insecticide-treated clothing, are the primary means of protection against vector-borne diseases. These personal protective measures should be recommended to all travelers visiting endemic areas. Air conditioning and well-screened rooms also should be used, especially if ITNs are not available. Although DEET is the most studied insect repellent available, picaridin, IR3535, and PMD are also efficacious. IR3535 is less effective against the *Anopheles* mosquito and should not be recommended to travelers visiting malaria-endemic regions. The combination of topical insect repellents and permethrin-treated clothing is ideal, offering near complete protection against arthropod bites. Finally, mosquito coils, vaporizers, essential oil candles, and insecticide knockdown sprays may prevent nuisance biting; however, not enough evidence exists for their use as a primary means of arthropod protection, especially in malaria and other endemic areas.

More research is needed in the area of arthropod protection measures. Poor traveler compliance and the developing resistance to insecticides remind us of the need for improvements to our current methods of protection, and for research into alternative methods that are user-friendly, affordable, and effective.

REFERENCES

1. Freedman DO, Weld LH, Kozarsky PE, et al. Spectrum of disease and relation to place of exposure among ill returned travelers. N Engl J Med 2006;354:119–30.
2. Leder K, Torresi J, Libman MD, et al. GeoSentinel surveillance of illness in returned travelers, 2007-2011. Ann Intern Med 2013;158:456–68.
3. Medlock JM, Leach SA. Effect of climate change on vector-borne disease risk in the UK. Lancet Infect Dis 2015;15:721–30.
4. Staple JE, Fischer M. Chikungunya virus in the Americas–what a vectorborne pathogen can do. N Engl J Med 2014;371:887–9.
5. Schoepke A, Steffen R, Gratz N. Effectiveness of personal protection measures against mosquito bites for malaria prophylaxis in travelers. J Travel Med 1998; 5:188–92.
6. Schlagenhauf P, Weld L, Goorhuis A, et al. Travel-associated infection presenting in Europe (2008–12): an analysis of EuroTravNet longitudinal, surveillance data,

and evaluation of the effect of the pre-travel consultation. Lancet Infect Dis 2015; 15:55–63.
7. Goodyer L, Song J. Mosquito bite-avoidance attitudes and behaviors in travelers at risk of malaria. J Travel Med 2014;21:33–8.
8. Heywood AE, Zhang M, MacIntyre CR, et al. Travel risk behaviours and uptake of pre-travel health preventions by university students in Australia. BMC Infect Dis 2012;12:43.
9. Barnett ED, MacPherson DW, Stauffer WM, et al. The visiting friends or relatives traveler in the 21st century: time for a new definition. J Travel Med 2010;17: 163–70.
10. Leder K, Tong S, Weld L, et al. Illness in travelers visiting friends and relatives: a review of the GeoSentinel Surveillance Network. Clin Infect Dis 2006;43:1185–93.
11. Bacaner N, Stauffer B, Boulware DR, et al. Travel medicine considerations for North American immigrants visiting friends and relatives. JAMA 2004;291: 2856–64.
12. Safaris W. ATTA Values Statement. 2013. Available at: http://www.adventuretravel.biz/wp-content/uploads/2013/02/Value-Statement-Consumer-English.pdf. Accessed August 9, 2015.
13. Herbinger KH, Siess C, Nothdurft HD, et al. Skin disorders among travellers returning from tropical and non-tropical countries consulting a travel medicine clinic. Trop Med Int Health 2011;16:1457–64.
14. Fournier PE, Roux V, Caumes E, et al. Outbreak of *Rickettsia africae* infections in participants of an adventure race in South Africa. Clin Infect Dis 1998;27: 316–23.
15. Pavli A, Maltezou HC. Leishmaniasis, an emerging infection in travelers. Int J Infect Dis 2010;14:e1032–9.
16. Centers for Disease Control and Prevention (CDC). Tick-borne encephalitis among US travelers to Europe and Asia—2000–2009. MMWR Morb Mortal Wkly Rep 2010;59:321–6.
17. Jensenius M, Fournier P-E, Vene S, et al. African tick bite fever in travelers to rural sub-Equatorial Africa. Clin Infect Dis 2003;36:1411–7.
18. Simarro PP, Franco JR, Cecchi G, et al. Human African trypanosomiasis in non-endemic countries (2000-2010). J Travel Med 2012;19:44–53.
19. Nasci RS, Wirtz RA, Brogdon WG. Protection against mosquitoes, ticks, & other arthropods. Centers for Disease Control and Prevention. CDC Health Information for International Travel 2016. New York: Oxford University Press; 2016.
20. Moore SJ, Mordue Luntz AJ, Logan JG. Insect bite prevention. Infect Dis Clin North Am 2012;26:655–73.
21. Dame DA, Meisch MV, Lewis CN, et al. Field evaluation of four spatial repellent devices against Arkansas rice-land mosquitoes. J Am Mosq Control Assoc 2014;30:31–6.
22. Ogoma SB, Moore SJ, Maia MF. A systematic review of mosquito coils and passive emanators: defining recommendations for spatial repellency testing methodologies. Parasit Vectors 2012;5:287.
23. Allan SA, Day JF, Edman JD. Visual ecology of biting flies. Annu Rev Entomol 1987;32:297–316.
24. Brun R, Blum J, Chappuis F, et al. Human African trypanosomiasis. Lancet 2010; 375:148–59.
25. Kline DL, Hogsette JA, Müller GC. Comparison of various configurations of CDC-type traps for the collection of *Phlebotomus papatasi Scopoli* in southern Israel. J Vector Ecol 2011;36:212–8.

26. Stanczyk NM, Behrens RH, Chen-Hussey V. Mosquito repellents for travellers case scenario. BMJ 2015;350:h99.
27. Goodyer LI, Croft AM, Frances SP, et al. Expert review of the evidence base for arthropod bite avoidance. J Travel Med 2010;17:182–92.
28. Osimitz TG, Murphy JV, Fell LA, et al. Adverse events associated with the use of insect repellents containing N,N-diethyl-m-toluamide (DEET). Regul Toxicol Pharmacol 2010;56:93–9.
29. Kitchen LW, Lawrence KL, Coleman RE. The role of the United States military in the development of vector control products, including insect repellents, insecticides, and bed nets. J Vector Ecol 2009;34:50–61.
30. Bohbot JD, Fu L, Le TC, et al. Multiple activities of insect repellents on odorant receptors in mosquitoes. Med Vet Entomol 2011;25:436–44.
31. Guidelines for testing: World Health Organization. Available at: http://whqlibdoc.who.int/hq/2009/WHO_HTM_NTD_WHOPES_2009.4_eng.pdf. Accessed August 9, 2015.
32. Fight the Bite for Protection against Malaria. Available at: http://www.cdc.gov/malaria/toolkit/DEET.pdf. Accessed August 7, 2015.
33. Lupi E, Hatz C, Schlagenhauf P. The efficacy of repellents against *Aedes, Anopheles, Culex* and *Ixodes* spp. – a literature review. Travel Med Infect Dis 2013;11:374–411.
34. Carroll JF, Benante JP, Klun JA, et al. Twelve-hour duration testing of cream formulations of three repellents against *Amblyomma americanum*. Med Vet Entomol 2008;22:144–51.
35. Dé F, Pages R, Dautel H, et al. Tick repellents for human use: prevention of tick bites and tick-borne diseases. Vector Borne Zoonotic Dis 2014;14:85–91.
36. Bohbot JD, Dickens JC. Insect repellents: modulators of mosquito odorant receptor activity. PLoS One 2010;5:e12138.
37. Van Roey K, Sokny M, Denis L, et al. Field evaluation of picaridin repellents reveals differences in repellent sensitivity between Southeast Asian vectors of malaria and arboviruses. PLoS Negl Trop Dis 2014;8:e3326.
38. Katz TM, Miller JH, Hebert AA. Insect repellents: historical perspectives and new developments. J Am Acad Dermatol 2008;58:865–70.
39. Chen-Hussey V, Behrens R, Logan JG. Assessment of methods used to determine the safety of the topical insect repellent N,N-diethyl-m-toluamide (DEET). Parasit Vectors 2014;7:173.
40. McGready R, Hamilton KA, Simpson JA, et al. Safety of the insect repellent N, N-diethyl-m-toluamide (DEET) in pregnancy. Am J Trop Med Hyg 2001;65: 285–9.
41. Banks SD, Murray N, Wilder-Smith A, et al. Insecticide-treated clothes for the control of vector-borne diseases: a review on effectiveness and safety. Med Vet Entomol 2014;28:14–25.
42. Gimnig JE, Vulule JM, Lo TQ, et al. Impact of permethrin-treated bed nets on entomologic indices in an area of intense year-round malaria transmission. Am J Trop Med Hyg 2003;68:16–22.
43. Gubler DJ. The continuing spread of West Nile virus in the western hemisphere. Clin Infect Dis 2007;45(8):1039–46.
44. Gershman MD, Staples JE. Chapter 3: Infectious diseases related to travel: yellow fever. Centers for Disease Control and Prevention. CDC Health Information for International Travel 2016. New York: Oxford University Press; 2016.
45. Hills SL, Rabe IB, Fischer M. Chapter 3: Infectious diseases related to Travel: Japanese Encephalitis. Centers for Disease Control and Prevention. CDC Health

Information for International Travel 2016. New York: Oxford University Press; 2016.
46. Herwaldt BL, Magill AJ. Chapter 3: Infectious diseases related to travel: leishmaniasis, cutaneous. Centers for Disease Control and Prevention. CDC Health Information for International Travel 2016. New York: Oxford University Press; 2016.
47. Centers for Disease Control - leishmaniasis - epidemiology and risk factors. Available at: http://www.cdc.gov/parasites/leishmaniasis/epi.html. Accessed August 9, 2015.
48. McQuiston J. Chapter 3: Rickettsial (spotted and typhus fevers) and related infections (anaplasmosis & ehrlichiosis). Centers for Disease Control and Prevention. CDC Health Information for International Travel 2016. New York: Oxford University Press; 2016.
49. Carroll SP. Prolonged efficacy of IR3535 repellents against mosquitoes and blacklegged ticks in North America. J Med Entomol 2008;45:706–14.

Traveler's Diarrhea

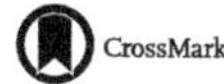

Stanley L. Giddings, MD[a], A. Michal Stevens, MD, MPH[a], Daniel T. Leung, MD, MSc[a,b,*]

KEYWORDS

• Travel • Diarrhea • Risk factors • Epidemiology • Antibiotic prophylaxis • Probiotics

KEY POINTS

- Traveler's diarrhea (TD) is the most common travel-related illness.
- Pretravel consultation is an opportunity to provide the traveler with education and therapeutic options to decrease the incidence and impact of TD.
- Early self-treatment of TD is effective, although its use must be balanced by consideration of medication side effects, acquisition of antimicrobial-resistant organisms through disturbance of gut flora, and potential for *Clostridium difficile* infection.
- Postinfectious sequelae of TD may result in presentation for care weeks or months after return from travel.

INTRODUCTION

More than 68 million Americans traveled abroad in 2014,[1] and the annual number of international tourist arrivals worldwide has reached more than 1 billion.[2] In data collected by GeoSentinel, a global surveillance network of international travelers, acute diarrhea was the most common among travel-related diagnostic groupings.[3] In this article, the epidemiology, cause, and strategies to prevent and treat traveler's diarrhea (TD) are reviewed.

Definition, Incidence, and Risk Factors

TD is defined as the passage of 3 or more unformed stools per day with 1 or more associated enteric symptom, such as abdominal pain or cramps, occurring in a traveler after arrival, usually in a resource-limited destination.[4]

[a] Division of Infectious Diseases, Department of Medicine, University of Utah School of Medicine, 30 North 1900 East, Salt Lake City, UT 84132, USA; [b] Division of Microbiology & Immunology, Department of Pathology, University of Utah School of Medicine, 15 North Medical Drive East, Salt Lake City, UT 84112, USA

* Corresponding author. Division of Infectious Diseases, University of Utah School of Medicine, 30 North 1900 East, SOM Room 4C416B, Salt Lake City, UT 84132.

E-mail address: Daniel.leung@utah.edu

Med Clin N Am 100 (2016) 317–330
http://dx.doi.org/10.1016/j.mcna.2015.08.017 medical.theclinics.com
0025-7125/16/$ – see front matter

Recent studies have shown that approximately 25% of travelers develop TD in the first 2 weeks abroad, with the highest rates occurring in travel to Africa and South, Central, and West Asia.[5,6] Factors that influence the incidence of TD vary based on the study design and location (**Table 1**).[5–7]

Cause

TD is predominantly a fecal-orally transmitted disease and can be caused by bacterial, viral, or protozoal pathogens, with helminths being uncommon. Many of the causes for TD (**Table 2**) are similar to those causing acute diarrhea in young children of low- and middle-income countries.[8] The frequency of each pathogen varies by geographic location, and the cause may be unknown in 40% to 50% of cases despite microbiologic evaluation,[9,10] although with increasing use of multiplex molecular testing,[11] this will likely change. Globally, enterotoxigenic *Escherichia coli* (ETEC) and enteroaggregative *E coli* (EAEC) are the most common bacterial pathogens,[9] with the exception of Southeast Asia, where *Campylobacter* is more common, a high proportion of which are fluoroquinolone resistant.[9,12] Norovirus and rotavirus are the most common viral causes of TD. Of the protozoa, *Giardia duodenalis* and *Entamoeba histolytica* are the main pathogens considered, depending on the region of travel. In some instances, TD may be due to more than one pathogen.

Impact on the Traveler

The median duration of TD is 3 days, and symptoms are usually mild, with approximately 4 bowel movements per day.[13] Unfortunately, TD can lead to significant limitation of activity. This incapacity typically lasts for 1 to 2 days,[14] resulting in loss of vacation or business days,[6] although data from one posttravel survey suggest that the majority with TD do not need to alter their planned programs.[15] Approximately 10% of travelers with TD seek medical care, and up to 3% of them require hospitalization.[14,16]

PRETRAVEL PREPARATION

The goals of pretravel consultation are to identify travelers at increased risk of travel-related illness and provide counseling, vaccinations, and medications for prophylaxis or self-treatment. Application of these principles at a pretravel consultation may decrease the incidence of TD.

Prevention

Impact of food and water hygiene measures

Given that most cases of TD are caused by ingestion of contaminated food and water, it is thought that counseling on food and water hygiene measures reduces the risk of TD. However, there is little evidence that such precautions decrease the incidence of

Table 1
Risk factors for traveler's diarrhea

Host-related factors	Country of origin (higher incidence if the traveler is from a highly industrialized country) Age (higher incidence in young adults 15–30)
Travel-related factors	Destination (higher incidence in travel to Africa and South, Central, and West Asia) Duration of stay (incidence increases until day 12 or day 14)

Data from Refs.[5–7]

Table 2
Causes of traveler's diarrhea

Pathogen	Organisms	Comments
Bacteria	ETEC EAEC *Campylobacter* spp *Shigella* spp *Salmonella* spp Enteropathogenic *E coli* *Aeromonas* spp *Plesiomonas shigelloides* *Vibrio* spp Enterotoxigenic *Bacteroides fragilis* *Acrobacter butzleri*	Southeast Asia has high prevalence of fluoroquinolone-resistant campylobacter isolates
Viral	Norovirus Rotavirus Astrovirus Sapovirus Adenovirus 40/41	Norovirus is associated with outbreaks on cruise ships
Protozoa	*G duodenalis* *Cryptosporidium parvum* *E histolytica* *Cyclospora cayetanensis* *Dientamoeba fragilis*	—
Unknown	No organism identified	Up to 50% of cases
Multiple pathogens	2 or more pathogens identified	Not uncommon, varying prevalence

Data from Shah N, DuPont HL, Ramsey DJ. Global etiology of travelers' diarrhea: systematic review from 1973 to the present. Am J Trop Med Hyg 2009;80(4):609–14; and Jiang ZD, Dupont HL, Brown EL, et al. Microbial etiology of travelers' diarrhea in Mexico, Guatemala, and India: importance of enterotoxigenic Bacteroides fragilis and Arcobacter species. J Clin Microbiol 2010;48(4):1417–19.

TD,[6,17] and it is likely that factors outside of a traveler's control, such as poor restaurant hygiene, may have a higher impact.[17] Despite this, travelers should be educated on appropriate food and water precautions (**Table 3**),[18] including frequent hand washing with soap.

Vaccines

There are no vaccines available against TD in the United States at this time. The oral killed whole-cell cholera vaccine, Dukoral, which is available in Canada and Europe, contains a recombinant cholera toxin B subunit, which is homologous with the heat-labile toxin (LT) of ETEC and by extension provides partial protection against TD. Unfortunately, worldwide, only approximately 25% of ETEC strains are LT-only (most express or coexpress the heat-stable toxin).[19] In a recent nonrandomized evaluation, the vaccine was found to provide 28% protection against TD.[20] Several vaccine candidates against ETEC are in various phases of development, including consideration of a combined ETEC/*Shigella* vaccine, targeting both travelers and children living in endemic countries.[21]

Probiotics

The use of probiotics for the prevention of TD is controversial and suffers from a lack of well-controlled studies. The challenges with using probiotic products include the

Table 3
Food and water precautions

High-Risk Foods	Strategies to Avoid High-Risk Foods
Salads	Consume peeled fruits and vegetables
Uncooked meat, fish, or eggs	Consume cooked food
Unpasteurized dairy products	Consume pasteurized dairy products
Tap or well water Products made using tap water or well water, such as ice or juice	Consume water that is bottled and sealed or water that is disinfected (boiled, filtered, treated)
Food from street vendors	Be wary of food and water hygiene at eating establishment
Food served at room temperature	Ensure meals are piping hot before consumption

Data from Centers for Disease Control and Prevention. Food and water safety. Available at: http://wwwnc.cdc.gov/travel/page/food-water-safety. Accessed June 26, 2015.

diversity of probiotic strains, the need for adequate quality control of products, defined optimal dose and duration of therapy, and specific storage requirements of some products. Attempts at systematic review of available studies have produced mixed results. One pooled meta-analysis of 12 randomized controlled trials showed that probiotics may be safe and effective at preventing TD,[22] with *Saccharomyces boulardii* and a mixture of *Lactobacillus acidophilus* and *Bifidobacterium bifidum* found to be efficacious. A subsequent review found that *S boulardii* afforded a dose-related protection for travelers to North Africa and *Lactobacillus rhamnosus strain GG* provided 12% to 45% protection against TD.[23] In contrast, a meta-analysis that reviewed 5 randomized controlled trials did not find any benefit from probiotic use.[24] More data are needed before definitive recommendations can be made on the use of probiotics for the prevention of TD.

Bismuth subsalicylate

Bismuth subsalicyclate (BSS) has been shown to provide up to 65% protection against TD when taken as 2 tablets 4 times per day for a maximum of 3 weeks.[25] It is usually well tolerated in young healthy adults. However, clinicians must warn travelers about blackening of the stool or tongue when taking this drug. BSS can decrease absorption of doxycycline, which may be used concomitantly for malaria prophylaxis.[26] A careful review of the traveler's medication list should be performed to look for potential drug-drug interactions. Although BSS provides moderate protection against TD, the need for frequent administration decreases the overall compliance and makes it a less attractive choice for most travelers.

Antibiotic chemoprophylaxis

Antibiotic chemoprophylaxis can provide up to 90% protection against TD.[27] Fluoroquinolones are effective prophylactic agents, and they provide a broad spectrum of activity against many common travel-related enteropathogens, including ETEC and EAEC. In a meta-analysis, they were shown to provide 88% protection against TD.[27] However, the risks of long-term quinolone therapy, including tendon rupture (especially in those with pre-existing kidney disease or on systemic corticosteroids), QTc prolongation, and *Clostridium difficile* infection, limit their usefulness as prophylaxis and should be discussed with the traveler.

Prophylactic rifaximin can provide up to 77% protection against TD,[28] although its effectiveness in Southeast Asia is lower (48% efficacy).[29] It is poorly absorbed from the gastrointestinal tract, and thus, systemic side effects are rare. However, rifaximin has poor activity against many enteroinvasive pathogens, and this is reflected in its decreased efficacy in SE.[29] Thus, the potential need for use of a second antimicrobial agent in the case of invasive disease, as well as its high cost relative to quinolones (**Table 4**), makes rifaximin a less attractive candidate.

For travelers to areas of Southeast Asia where there are high rates of quinolone resistance, it is reasonable to consider prophylaxis with azithromycin, but there are minimal data for its use in travelers; the safety of prophylactic use of azithromycin is extrapolated from studies in cystic fibrosis and HIV (human immunodeficiency virus) patients.

The advantages and efficacy of antibiotic prophylaxis are tempered by the risks of side effects, *C difficile* infection, acquisition of antimicrobial-resistant organisms, and cost. Thus, the authors recommend that its use be reserved only for high-risk travelers such as those who are immunosuppressed or those in whom an episode of TD may lead to increased morbidity.[27] Although chemoprophylaxis may also be considered in travelers with little flexible time, such as politicians, athletes, or performers, early self-treatment (see later discussion) may be more appropriate.

Traveler-Initiated Symptomatic Treatment

Self-treatment on initial symptoms is the mainstay of TD management, the backbone of which is oral rehydration therapy. Adding to that backbone, for mild cases, the use of bismuth and loperamide is effective and sufficient. For moderate or severe TD, the use of empiric oral antibiotics has been found to be effective in shortening the duration of symptoms, although there is increasing evidence that this practice may have societal and personal health costs.

Oral rehydration

Adequate oral fluid intake is essential to both prevent and treat dehydration related to TD. For mild dehydration, simply increasing the amount of oral fluid intake with clean water or readily available fluids is adequate. For moderate or severe dehydration, and particularly in children, elderly, and those with chronic medical conditions, the authors recommend World Health Organization–formulated oral rehydration salts (ORS),[30] which have been shown to be similar in efficacy as intravenous fluids in children presenting to a US emergency room.[31] ORS can be prepared at home (**Box 1**),[32] or it is available as packaged commercial products sold in pharmacies and stores worldwide. Commonly used beverages, such as Gatorade, apple juice, or soft drinks, may not be appropriate for repletion of moderate or severe dehydration because of their high-sugar and low-salt content, although data comparing their use with ORS are lacking.

Antidiarrheal medication

Loperamide is safe and effective for treatment of nondysenteric TD.[33] It can be used alone for mild cases and as an adjunct with antibiotics (see later discussion) for

Table 4
Chemoprophylaxis options for traveler's diarrhea

Drug	Dosing	Average Cost for a 2-wk Trip[a]
Bismuth	2 tablets qid	$14.56
Ciprofloxacin	500 mg daily	$44.52
Rifaximin	200 mg daily or bid	$246.96–$493.92

[a] Cost is based on average wholesale price.

Box 1
Recipe for oral rehydration salt

½ teaspoon of salt + 6 level teaspoons of sugar + 1 L of safe water (water that is bottled and sealed or disinfected)

OR

Lightly salted rice water

Data from World Health Organization. WHO position paper on oral rehydration salts to reduce mortality from cholera. Available at: http://www.who.int/cholera/technical/en/. Accessed July 1, 2015.

moderate or severe TD. A meta-analysis found that compared with antibiotic therapy alone, adjunctive loperamide decreased the duration of illness and increased the probability of cure.[33]

Apart from BSS being used to prevent TD, it can also be used to treat TD. It has been shown to reduce the passage of unformed stools, and it may be useful for the treatment of mild TD.[34] However, when compared with loperamide, it has a delayed onset of action and is less effective, with estimates of loperamide providing more than 50% reduction in passage of unformed stools compared with BSS providing a 16% to 18% reduction.[34]

Early antibiotic self-treatment

Early self-treatment of TD with antibiotic therapy has been shown to be effective at reducing the duration of symptoms.[35] In a randomized placebo-controlled trial, early self-treatment of TD with ciprofloxacin reduced the duration of symptoms from 81 to 29 hours.[35] The authors recommend offering travelers a prescription of antibiotics for early self-treatment, but emphasizing its use only for moderate to severe TD and for dysentery. Antibiotics can be given as a single-dose regimen or as a multiple-dose regimen for up to 3 days (**Table 5**). For travelers on the multiple-dose regimens, if the symptoms resolve after 1 or 2 doses, the antibiotic therapy can be stopped.

The antibiotic agent selected should be tailored to the region of travel and the prevalence of multi-drug-resistant pathogens in that region. Either ciprofloxacin or rifaximin may be used for most global destinations, but travelers to South and Southeast Asia should receive azithromycin, given the high incidence of quinolone-resistant enteropathogens.[12] Rifaximin use is often limited by cost. Notably, azithromycin and levofloxacin (although not ciprofloxacin) have been associated with increased risk of ventricular arrhythmia and cardiovascular death,[36] and given the risk of electrolyte imbalances during severe diarrhea, a high level of caution should be used when

Table 5
Antibiotic self-treatment options for traveler's diarrhea in healthy adults

Drug	Dosing	Average Cost for 3 d of Therapy[a]
Azithromycin	500 mg daily × 3 d or 1 g single dose	\$25.32–\$46.71
Ciprofloxacin	500 mg bid × 3 d or 750 mg single dose	\$19.08
Rifaximin	200 mg 3 times daily × 3 d	\$158.76

[a] Cost is based on average wholesale price.

prescribing these agents in patients with pre-existing heart disease, and should be avoided in those with known QT prolongation.

Several recent reports have associated the use of antibiotics for TD with an increased risk of acquisition of extended-spectrum β-lactamase (ESBL) Enterobacteriaceae organisms.[37,38] Although the persistence of ESBL colonization in returning travelers appears to be relatively short, and no infection has been directly linked to such colonization, the long-term societal and personal health consequences are not known. Thus, the authors recommend education and discussions regarding appropriate use of antibiotics, including mention of the self-resolving nature of most cases of TD, and the risks associated with antibiotic use, including their side effects, *C difficile* infection, and acquisition of multidrug-resistant bacteria. Other factors to be considered are the availability of appropriate medical care, and the safety and purity of antibiotics, in the destination country.

When to seek medical care

A TD pretravel kit (**Box 2**) is a useful tool that can limit the duration of TD and its impact on the traveler. Travelers should be encouraged to carry this kit during their trip, and they should be counseled on how to use it effectively. However, they should seek medical care for persistent fever, chills, bloody diarrhea, moderate to severe abdominal pain, intractable vomiting, if they are unable to retain oral fluid intake, or if their symptoms worsen or persist despite early self-treatment. Special traveler populations are more at risk for severe and complicated TD, and these travelers should have a low threshold to seek medical attention. Information on clinics in destination countries specializing in travel medicine can be obtained from the International Society of Travel Medicine (http://www.istm.org/AF_CstmClinicDirectory.asp) or the International Association for Medical Assistance to Travellers (https://www.iamat.org).

SPECIAL POPULATIONS

Pregnant Women

Pregnant women may be more prone to TD due to reduced gastric acidity and slowed intestinal motility.[39] In one study, TD occurred in 11% of pregnant travelers to developing countries.[40] The main pretravel advice for pregnant women are counseling on food and water hygiene as well as ensuring adequate fluid hydration.[39] Antimicrobial chemoprophylaxis is not recommended for pregnant travelers. Clinicians must be wary of medication use and their potential for adverse pregnancy outcome, fetal harm, and secretion of medications into breast milk. BSS and fluoroquinolones are not recommended in pregnancy, and loperamide and rifaximin are pregnancy class C drugs. Azithromycin, which is pregnancy class B, is the drug of choice for early self-treatment of TD.

Box 2
Traveler's diarrhea pretravel kit

- Instructions on food safety and water hygiene
- ORS recipe
- Antidiarrheal medication (loperamide)
- Self-treatment antibiotics (fluoroquinolone, azithromycin, or rifaximin) with instructions on use OR antimicrobial chemoprophylaxis for select travelers
- Emergency medical contacts locally and abroad

Children

Infants and young children with TD have a more severe and prolonged course of disease and are more likely to present with fever and bloody diarrhea.[41,42] The mainstay of treatment is rehydration, and parents should be advised on appropriate oral rehydration solution. Antimicrobial chemoprophylaxis, loperamide, and BSS are usually not recommended for this population, and parents should have a low threshold to seek medical care if the child develops bloody diarrhea, fever with temperature greater than 101.5°F, moderate to severe dehydration, or persistent vomiting, or for any changes in mental status. For antibiotic self-treatment, azithromycin is the drug of choice.[42] Although trimethoprim/sulfamethoxazole has been used in the past, because of increasing resistance worldwide, the authors recommend cefixime or other third-generation cephalosporins as second-line agents, although they may be ineffective against campylobacter.[43] Fluoroquinolones are not recommended in children less than 18 years of age because of the potential for cartilage damage based on animal studies. There is ongoing review on the safety of this drug in children, and it may have a role in targeted treatment of multidrug-resistant enteropathogens.[44]

Immunocompromised Host

The immunocompromised host would benefit from a multidisciplinary evaluation before travel so that travel-related issues including prevention and management of TD can be discussed.[45] Antimicrobial chemoprophylaxis for TD should be considered,[45] although there is increased potential for drug-drug interactions in this population. Immunocompromised host travelers also need to have a contingency plan in case of a medical emergency; this plan should include medical contact both locally and abroad.

Comorbid Disease

Travelers with comorbid disease, such as insulin-dependent diabetes mellitus, heart failure, or renal insufficiency, may not be able to tolerate an episode of TD, because it can lead to severe electrolyte imbalance and dehydration with subsequent exacerbation of their underlying medical condition. The importance of ensuring adequate hydration must be stressed to these travelers. Antimicrobial chemoprophylaxis and early self-treatment options must be discussed in relation to their comorbidities and careful attention to their home medication list, and potential drug-drug interactions must be noted. The risk of ventricular arrhythmia and cardiovascular death with azithromycin and levofloxacin is an important consideration.[36]

POSTTRAVEL MANAGEMENT

TD can occur, or persist, after the traveler has returned home. The time to onset of symptoms would depend on the incubation period of the pathogen. Typically this would be up to 2 weeks after return from travel, but this incubation period may be longer when protozoa or helminths are the etiologic agents.

Persistent Diarrhea After Travel

Infectious gastrointestinal disease accounts for approximately 30% of diagnoses of returning travelers who present for medical care.[46] Common pathogens associated with diarrheal illness in returned travelers include bacterial causes with longer incubation periods (such as *Campylobacter*, *Shigella*, *Salmonella*), protozoa (Giardia, cryptosporidium, cyclospora, *E histolytica*, and *Dientamoeba fragilis*), as well as helminthes such as Ascaris, Strongyloides, and hookworms. In particular, if there is a history of antibiotic use, *C difficile* infection should also be considered.[47]

Evaluation

A detailed history and physical examination should be performed in all travelers seeking medical care for diarrhea on return home. This examination should include information on areas visited during their trip and specific exposures that may provide clues to the cause. Drug-resistant pathogens must also be considered, taking into account the region of travel and prior antibiotic therapy.

Consultation with a travel medicine expert may be useful and workup may include a complete blood count with differential (eosinophilia may suggest helminthic infection), and stool for microscopy (ova and parasites), and antigen-based testing. *C difficile* testing may also be warranted. Serologic investigation for *Strongyloides* and *Schistosoma* may also be obtained when clinically indicated. Recent advances in molecular diagnostics have led to the development and marketing of several stool multiplex polymerase chain reaction (PCR) panels for gastrointestinal pathogens (**Table 6**). There is a lack of published studies examining the utility of such panels in returning travelers, although there may be benefits with respect to their sensitivity, cost-effectiveness, and timeliness, compared with traditional methods. However, results from such panels in returning travelers need to be interpreted with caution, given the likelihood of multiple pathogens identified.

Postinfectious Sequelae

Postinfectious irritable bowel syndrome

Travel-associated diarrhea afflicts a relatively large proportion of international travelers, and the majority experience complete recovery without further symptoms. In some, however, despite clearance of the infectious pathogen from the gut, there is persistence or recurrence of abdominal symptoms, similar to that described for irritable bowel syndrome (IBS).[48,49] It is unclear whether the pathogenesis of travel-related IBS, especially that experienced by long-term travelers,[48] is the same as that of non-travel-associated postinfectious irritable bowel syndrome (PI-IBS). Possible mechanisms include a reversible small intestinal enteropathy, such as described in the 1970s in Peace Corp volunteers returning from Pakistan,[50] also known as tropical enteropathy in residents of low-income countries,[51] tropical sprue, or the unmasking of an underlying gastrointestinal disorder.[52] Nevertheless, many patients do meet Rome III diagnostic criteria for IBS, and overall, approximately 3% to 20% of travelers develop PI-IBS, with most cases being diarrhea-predominant.

Known risk factors for developing PI-IBS include duration of initial illness, severity of initial illness, smoking, degree of gut inflammation, female gender, and presence of stress at the time of the initial illness.[53] Gulf War Veterans in particular seem to have an increased risk of developing PI-IBS.[54]

It is possible that treatment modalities commonly used for TD, such as antibiotics and antimotility agents, may not only alter the course of TD but also impact its potential to develop PI-IBS. However, these associations are poorly understood and not well studied. Despite recent studies showing the efficacy of rifaximin for IBS,[55] it has not been evaluated in PI-IBS, and at this point, the authors do not recommend its use in returning travelers. Further investigation into the microbiota and mucosal immune correlates of post-travel IBS is warranted.

Although the prognosis of posttravel PI-IBS is unknown, a recent study of post-Shigella IBS patients showed that roughly half of patients with PI-IBS recovered by 5 years after onset, and also that patients with a history of IBS before infection were more likely to have a prolonged course of illness beyond 5 years.[56]

Table 6
Comparison of pathogens tested by various multiplex polymerase chain reactions

	FilmArray Gastrointestinal Panel (BioFire Diagnostics, Inc, Salt Lake City, UT, USA)	xTag Gastrointestinal Pathogen Panel (Luminex Corporation, Austin, TX, USA)	Verigene Enteric Pathogen Test (Nanosphere, Northbrook, IL, USA)
Bacteria and bacterial toxins			
Campylobacter spp[a]	x	x	x
Salmonella spp	x	x	x
Vibrio cholerae	x	—	—
Vibrio spp	x	—	x
Yersinia entercolitica	x	—	x
C difficile (toxin A/B)	x	x	—
Plesiomonas shigelloides	x	—	—
Enteroinvasive *E coli/Shigella* spp	x	x	x
E coli O157	x	x	—
Enterotoxigenic *E coli* (ETEC) lt/st	x	x	—
EAEC	x	—	—
Enteropathogenic *E coli* (EPEC)	x	—	—
Shiga toxin producing *E coli* (STEC) stx1/stx2	x	x	x
Viruses			
Adenovirus 40/41	x	—	—
Astrovirus	x	—	—
Norovirus	x	x	x
Rotavirus	x	x	x
Sapovirus (I, II, IV, and V)	x	—	—
Parasites			
Cryptosporidium	x	x	—
Cyclopora cayetanesis	x	—	—
E histolytica	x	—	—
Giardia lamblia	x	x	—

[a] *Campylobacter* spp varies with test performed.

Reactive arthritis

Reactive arthritis can occur 1 to 4 weeks after an episode of TD.[49,57] It is an oligoarthritis that is asymmetric and typically involves the lower limbs or sacroiliac joint. It can have an acute self-limited course lasting months or lead to chronic (refractory) symptoms for years.[49,57] Several TD pathogens, including *Shigella*, *Campylobacter*, *Salmonella*, and *E coli*, have been associated with reactive arthritis, and host factors such as HLA B27 are also implicated.[49]

Guillain-Barré syndrome

Guillain-Barré syndrome may also develop 1 to 4 weeks after a bout of TD.[49] The preceding enteric infection is usually due to *Campylobacter*, although other enteric gram-negative bacteria can trigger this phenomenon, in which an autoimmune response is mounted against peripheral nerves leading to peripheral neuropathy or acute neuromuscular failure.[49] There is a bimodal peak in incidence with young adults and the elderly most commonly affected. This disease can result in permanent disability or even death.

SUMMARY

TD is the most common travel-related illness. Pretravel consultation by the health care provider is an excellent opportunity to educate the traveler and provide them with resources to decrease the incidence and impact of the disease. Early self-treatment is an effective strategy for moderate to severe TD, although its benefits must be weighed against risks of adverse effects and acquisition of antimicrobial-resistant bacteria. Persistent diarrhea and postinfectious sequelae of TD can present after return from travel, and such travelers may benefit from specialist referral.

ACKNOWLEDGMENTS

The authors thank Dr Brian Kendall (University of Utah) for his helpful review of this article.

REFERENCES

1. U.S. Department of Commerce, International Trade Administration, National Travel and Tourism Office. U.S. Citizen Traffic to Overseas Regions, Canada & Mexico 2014. In: Monthly Statistics, U.S. Outbound Travel by World Regions. 2014. Available at: http://travel.trade.gov/view/m-2014-O-001/index.html. Accessed June 26, 2015.
2. The World Bank. World development indicators. In: Online tables, global links, 6.14 travel and tourism. Available at: http://wdi.worldbank.org/table/6.14. Accessed July 1, 2015.
3. Harvey K, Esposito DH, Han P, et al. Surveillance for travel-related disease–GeoSentinel Surveillance System, United States, 1997-2011. MMWR Surveill Summ 2013;62:1–23.
4. Dupont HL. For the record: a history of the definition & management of travelers' diarrhea. In: Yellow book, chapter 2, the pre-travel consultation. 2013. Available at: http://wwwnc.cdc.gov/travel/yellowbook/2014/chapter-2-the-pre-travel-consultation/for-the-record-a-history-of-the-definition-and-management-of-travelers-diarrhea. Accessed June 26, 2015.
5. Pitzurra R, Steffen R, Tschopp A, et al. Diarrhoea in a large prospective cohort of European travellers to resource-limited destinations. BMC Infect Dis 2010;10:231.
6. Lalani T, Maguire JD, Grant EM, et al. Epidemiology and self-treatment of travelers' diarrhea in a large, prospective cohort of department of defense beneficiaries. J Travel Med 2015;22(3):152–60.

7. Steffen R, Tornieporth N, Clemens SA, et al. Epidemiology of travelers' diarrhea: details of a global survey. J Travel Med 2004;11(4):231–7.
8. Kotloff KL, Nataro JP, Blackwelder WC, et al. Burden and aetiology of diarrhoeal disease in infants and young children in developing countries (the Global Enteric Multicenter Study, GEMS): a prospective, case-control study. Lancet 2013; 382(9888):209–22.
9. Shah N, DuPont HL, Ramsey DJ. Global etiology of travelers' diarrhea: systematic review from 1973 to the present. Am J Trop Med Hyg 2009;80(4):609–14.
10. Jiang ZD, Dupont HL, Brown EL, et al. Microbial etiology of travelers' diarrhea in Mexico, Guatemala, and India: importance of enterotoxigenic Bacteroides fragilis and Arcobacter species. J Clin Microbiol 2010;48(4):1417–9.
11. Khare R, Espy MJ, Cebelinski E, et al. Comparative evaluation of two commercial multiplex panels for detection of gastrointestinal pathogens by use of clinical stool specimens. J Clin Microbiol 2014;52(10):3667–73.
12. Tribble DR, Sanders JW, Pang LW, et al. Traveler's diarrhea in Thailand: randomized, double-blind trial comparing single-dose and 3-day azithromycin-based regimens with a 3-day levofloxacin regimen. Clin Infect Dis 2007; 44(3):338–46.
13. Steffen R, van der Linde F, Gyr K, et al. Epidemiology of diarrhea in travelers. JAMA 1983;249(9):1176–80.
14. von Sonnenburg F, Tornieporth N, Waiyaki P, et al. Risk and aetiology of diarrhoea at various tourist destinations. Lancet 2000;356(9224):133–4.
15. Soonawala D, Vlot JA, Visser LG. Inconvenience due to travelers' diarrhea: a prospective follow-up study. BMC Infect Dis 2011;11:322.
16. Piyaphanee W, Kusolsuk T, Kittitrakul C, et al. Incidence and impact of travelers' diarrhea among foreign backpackers in Southeast Asia: a result from Khao San road, Bangkok. J Travel Med 2011;18(2):109–14.
17. Shlim DR. Looking for evidence that personal hygiene precautions prevent traveler's diarrhea. Clin Infect Dis 2005;41(Suppl 8):S531–5.
18. Centers for Disease Control and Prevention. Food and water safety. In: Common travel health topics. 2013. Available at: http://wwwnc.cdc.gov/travel/page/food-water-safety. Accessed June 26, 2015.
19. Isidean SD, Riddle MS, Savarino SJ, et al. A systematic review of ETEC epidemiology focusing on colonization factor and toxin expression. Vaccine 2011;29(37): 6167–78.
20. Lopez-Gigosos R, Campins M, Calvo MJ, et al. Effectiveness of the WC/rBS oral cholera vaccine in the prevention of traveler's diarrhea: a prospective cohort study. Hum Vaccin Immunother 2013;9(3):692–8.
21. Walker RI, Clifford A. Recommendations regarding the development of combined enterotoxigenic Eschericha coli and Shigella vaccines for infants. Vaccine 2015; 33(8):946–53.
22. McFarland LV. Meta-analysis of probiotics for the prevention of traveler's diarrhea. Travel Med Infect Dis 2007;5(2):97–105.
23. DuPont HL, Ericsson CD, Farthing MJ, et al. Expert review of the evidence base for prevention of travelers' diarrhea. J Travel Med 2009;16(3):149–60.
24. Takahashi O, Noguchi Y, Omata F, et al. Probiotics in the prevention of traveler's diarrhea: meta-analysis. J Clin Gastroenterol 2007;41(3):336–7.
25. DuPont HL, Ericsson CD, Johnson PC, et al. Use of bismuth subsalicylate for the prevention of travelers' diarrhea. Rev Infect Dis 1990;12(Suppl 1):S64–7.
26. Ericsson CD, Feldman S, Pickering LK, et al. Influence of subsalicylate bismuth on absorption of doxycycline. JAMA 1982;247(16):2266–7.

27. Alajbegovic S, Sanders JW, Atherly DE, et al. Effectiveness of rifaximin and fluoroquinolones in preventing travelers' diarrhea (TD): a systematic review and meta-analysis. Syst Rev 2012;1:39.
28. DuPont HL, Jiang ZD, Okhuysen PC, et al. A randomized, double-blind, placebo-controlled trial of rifaximin to prevent travelers' diarrhea. Ann Intern Med 2005; 142(10):805–12.
29. Zanger P, Nurjadi D, Gabor J, et al. Effectiveness of rifaximin in prevention of diarrhoea in individuals travelling to south and southeast Asia: a randomised, double-blind, placebo-controlled, phase 3 trial. Lancet Infect Dis 2013;13(11):946–54.
30. King CK, Glass R, Bresee JS, et al. Managing acute gastroenteritis among children: oral rehydration, maintenance, and nutritional therapy. MMWR Recomm Rep 2003;52(RR–16):1–16.
31. Spandorfer PR, Alessandrini EA, Joffe MD, et al. Oral versus intravenous rehydration of moderately dehydrated children: a randomized, controlled trial. Pediatrics 2005;115(2):295–301.
32. World Health Organization. WHO position paper on Oral Rehydration Salts to reduce mortality from cholera. In: Global Task Force on Cholera Control. Available at: http://www.who.int/cholera/technical/en/. Accessed July 1, 2015.
33. Riddle MS, Arnold S, Tribble DR. Effect of adjunctive loperamide in combination with antibiotics on treatment outcomes in traveler's diarrhea: a systematic review and meta-analysis. Clin Infect Dis 2008;47(8):1007–14.
34. Ericsson CD. Nonantimicrobial agents in the prevention and treatment of traveler's diarrhea. Clin Infect Dis 2005;41(Suppl 8):S557–63.
35. Ericsson CD, Johnson PC, Dupont HL, et al. Ciprofloxacin or trimethoprim-sulfamethoxazole as initial therapy for travelers' diarrhea. A placebo-controlled, randomized trial. Ann Intern Med 1987;106(2):216–20.
36. Chou HW, Wang JL, Chang CH, et al. Risks of cardiac arrhythmia and mortality among patients using new-generation macrolides, fluoroquinolones, and beta-lactam/beta-lactamase inhibitors: a Taiwanese nationwide study. Clin Infect Dis 2015;60(4):566–77.
37. Kantele A, Laaveri T, Mero S, et al. Antimicrobials increase travelers' risk of colonization by extended-spectrum betalactamase-producing Enterobacteriaceae. Clin Infect Dis 2015;60(6):837–46.
38. Ruppe E, Armand-Lefevre L, Estellat C, et al. High rate of acquisition but short duration of carriage of multidrug-resistant enterobacteriaceae after travel to the tropics. Clin Infect Dis 2015;61(4):593–600.
39. Carroll ID, Williams DC. Pre-travel vaccination and medical prophylaxis in the pregnant traveler. Travel Med Infect Dis 2008;6(5):259–75.
40. Sammour RN, Bahous R, Grupper M, et al. Pregnancy course and outcome in women traveling to developing countries. J Travel Med 2012;19(5):289–93.
41. Pitzinger B, Steffen R, Tschopp A. Incidence and clinical features of traveler's diarrhea in infants and children. Pediatr Infect Dis J 1991;10(10):719–23.
42. Fox TG, Manaloor JJ, Christenson JC. Travel-related infections in children. Pediatr Clin North Am 2013;60(2):507–27.
43. Suh KN, Mileno MD. Challenging scenarios in a travel clinic: advising the complex traveler. Infect Dis Clin North Am 2005;19(1):15–47.
44. Bradley JS, Jackson MA, Committee on Infectious Diseases, American Academy of Pediatric. The use of systemic and topical fluoroquinolones. Pediatrics 2011; 128(4):e1034–1045.
45. Askling HH, Dalm VA. The medically immunocompromised adult traveler and pre-travel counseling: status quo 2014. Travel Med Infect Dis 2014;12(3):219–28.

46. Swaminathan A, Torresi J, Schlagenhauf P, et al. A global study of pathogens and host risk factors associated with infectious gastrointestinal disease in returned international travellers. J Infect 2009;59(1):19–27.
47. Neuberger A, Saadi T, Shetern A, et al. Clostridium difficile infection in travelers–a neglected pathogen? J Travel Med 2013;20(1):37–43.
48. Tuteja AK, Talley NJ, Gelman SS, et al. Development of functional diarrhea, constipation, irritable bowel syndrome, and dyspepsia during and after traveling outside the USA. Dig Dis Sci 2008;53(1):271–6.
49. Connor BA, Riddle MS. Post-infectious sequelae of travelers' diarrhea. J Travel Med 2013;20(5):303–12.
50. Lindenbaum J, Gerson CD, Kent TH. Recovery of small-intestinal structure and function after residence in the tropics. I. Studies in Peace Corps volunteers. Ann Intern Med 1971;74(2):218–22.
51. Veitch AM, Kelly P, Zulu IS, et al. Tropical enteropathy: a T-cell-mediated crypt hyperplastic enteropathy. Eur J Gastroenterol Hepatol 2001;13(10):1175–81.
52. Giannella RA. Chronic diarrhea in travelers: diagnostic and therapeutic considerations. Rev Infect Dis 1986;8(Suppl 2):S223–6.
53. Verdu EF, Riddle MS. Chronic gastrointestinal consequences of acute infectious diarrhea: evolving concepts in epidemiology and pathogenesis. Am J Gastroenterol 2012;107(7):981–9.
54. Trivedi KH, Schlett CD, Tribble DR, et al. The impact of post-infectious functional gastrointestinal disorders and symptoms on the health-related quality of life of US military personnel returning from deployment to the Middle East. Dig Dis Sci 2011;56(12):3602–9.
55. Iorio N, Malik Z, Schey R. Profile of rifaximin and its potential in the treatment of irritable bowel syndrome. Clin Exp Gastroenterol 2015;8:159–67.
56. Jung IS, Kim HS, Park H, et al. The clinical course of postinfectious irritable bowel syndrome: a five-year follow-up study. J Clin Gastroenterol 2009;43(6):534–40.
57. Yates JA, Stetz LC. Reiter's syndrome (reactive arthritis) and travelers' diarrhea. J Travel Med 2006;13(1):54–6.

Road Traffic and Other Unintentional Injuries Among Travelers to Developing Countries

Barclay T. Stewart, MD, MscPH[a,b,c,*], Isaac Kofi Yankson, MPH[d], Francis Afukaar, MSc[d], Martha C. Hijar Medina, PhD[e], Pham Viet Cuong, PhD[f], Charles Mock, MD, PhD[g,h,i,j,k]

KEYWORDS

- Road traffic injuries • Drowning • Burn • Fall • Unintentional injury
- Injury prevention • Travel medicine • Advocacy

KEY POINTS

- Road traffic crashes are the most common cause of travelers' deaths.
- Travelers can protect themselves and set an example by always wearing a seatbelt, never driving after consuming alcohol, and wearing a helmet when riding a motorcycle, moped, or bicycle.
- Drowning is the most common cause of death among travelers to water recreation destinations.

Continued

Funding: This study was funded by grants (R25-TW009345; D43-TW007267) from the Fogarty International Center, US National Institutes of Health. The content is solely the responsibility of the authors and does not necessarily represent the official views of the National Institutes of Health.
Disclosure Statement: No real or potential conflicts to disclose.
[a] Department of Surgery, University of Washington, 1959 Northeast Pacific Street, Suite BB-487, PO Box 356410, Seattle, WA 98195-6410, USA; [b] School of Medical Sciences, Kwame Nkrumah University of Science and Technology, Kumasi, Ghana; [c] Department of Surgery, Komfo Anokye Teaching Hospital, Kumasi, Ghana; [d] CSIR-Building and Road Research Institute, University PO Box 40, Kumasi, Ghana; [e] Secretaria Técnica del CONAPRA, Subsecretaría de Prevención y Promoción Secretaría Salud, Guadalajara 46 3er. Piso Col Roma Norte, CP 06700, Mexico DF, Mexico; [f] Center for Injury Policy and Prevention Research, Department of Public Health Informatics, Hanoi School of Public Health, 138 Giảng Võ, Kim Mã, Ba Đình, Hanoi, Vietnam; [g] Department of Surgery, University of Washington, Seattle, WA, USA; [h] Department of Epidemiology, University of Washington, Seattle, WA, USA; [i] Department of Global Health, University of Washington, Seattle, WA, USA; [j] Harborview Injury Prevention & Research Center, Patricia Bracelin Steel Memorial Building, 401 Broadway, 4th Floor, Seattle, WA 98122, USA; [k] Harborview Medical Center, 325 9th Avenue, Seattle, WA 98104, USA
* Corresponding author. Department of Surgery, University of Washington, 1959 Northeast Pacific Street, Suite BB-487, PO Box 356410, Seattle, WA 98195-6410.
E-mail address: stewarb@u.washington.edu

Med Clin N Am 100 (2016) 331–343
http://dx.doi.org/10.1016/j.mcna.2015.07.011 medical.theclinics.com

Continued

- Closely supervising children, wearing a personal flotation device, and practicing pool, open water, and boat safety can lower drowning risk.
- Advocacy is a way for travelers to make a difference that lasts long after their trip and for travel medicine providers to contribute to patient and population health more broadly.

INTRODUCTION

Injuries result in nearly 6 million deaths and incur 52 million disability-adjusted life-years annually, making up 15% of the global disease burden.[1] More than 90% of this burden occurs in low- and middle-income countries (LMICs) where injury control capacity and initiatives are lacking.[2] When trauma services do exist, they are often insufficiently resourced and unavailable to most of the injured.[3] Consequently, treatable injuries frequently result in avertable death or disability.[4]

Injuries are the leading cause of death among travelers.[5] Travelers abroad are 10 times more likely to die from injury than infection, accounting for less than 2% of traveler deaths.[6] Of traveler unintentional injuries, road traffic crashes account for 57% of deaths, followed by drowning (25%), aviation crashes (7%), other causes (eg, falls, burns; 6%), and natural disasters (4%) (**Fig. 1**).[7]

Despite high injury risk, pretravel advice has concentrated on communicable and vaccine-preventable diseases, such as malaria, typhoid, and diarrhea.[8] However, among individuals age 15 to 49 in LMICs (ie, same age cohort as 65% high-income country travelers), road traffic injuries (RTIs) alone are responsible for more deaths than these 3 diseases combined (**Fig. 2**).[7,9] A survey of travel medicine clinics worldwide found that 99% offered advice on infections; only 70% discussed personal safety.[10] Fortunately, nearly two-thirds of injuries are preventable.[11,12] Therefore, pretravel advice regarding foreseeable dangers and how to avoid them may significantly mitigate injury risk.[13] Pretravel consultations are incomplete without specific injury prevention advice.[11]

This article discusses the epidemiology, risk, and pretravel advice regarding road traffic injuries and drowning. Other causes of traveler injury, such as aviation crashes,

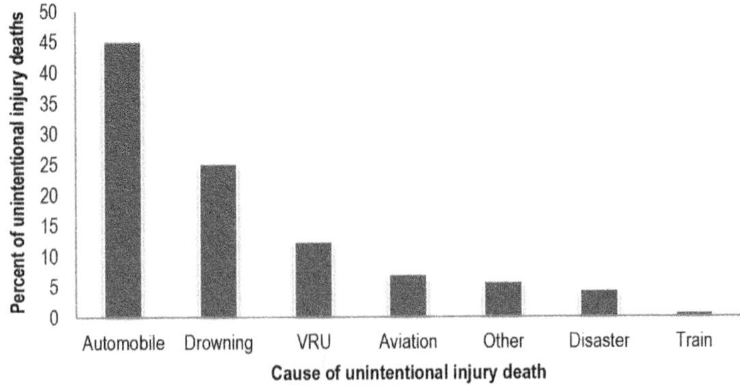

Fig. 1. Percentage of unintentional injury deaths by mechanism for US travelers from 2003 to 2014 (N = 4479). Unintentional injuries exclude homicide, suicide, and terrorism. VRU, Vulnerable road user. (*Data from* United States Department of State - Bureau of Consular Affairs. U.S. Citizen Deaths Overseas. Available at: http://travel.state.gov/content/travel/english/statistics/deaths.html. Accessed July 28, 2015.)

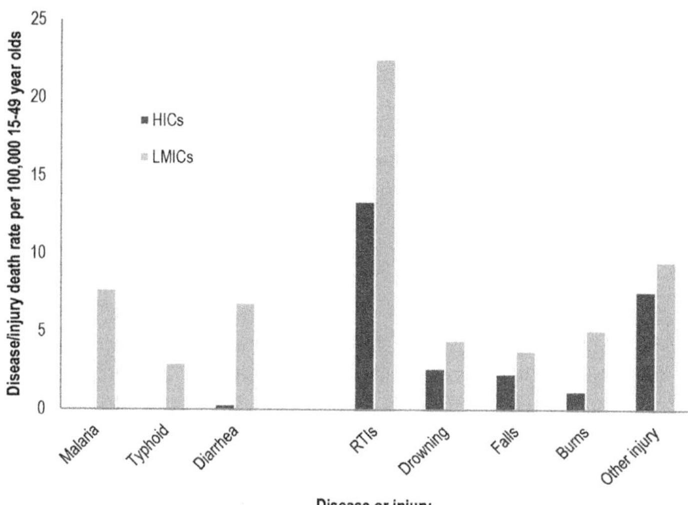

Fig. 2. Death rate per 100,000 15- to 49-year-olds for selected diseases and injuries in high-income and low- and middle-income countries. Other injury includes mechanical forces, non–road traffic transport injuries (eg, aviation crashes), animal contact. Age 15 to 49 years was selected, as it represents the same age cohort as 65% of HIC travelers. (*Data from* Institute of Health Metrics and Evaluation. GBD Cause Patterns. Available at: http://vizhub.healthdata.org/gbd-cause-patterns/. Accessed May 27, 2015.)

falls, burns, and those associated with adventure activities are also mentioned.[5] When returning, travelers to LMICs are in a unique position; having been exposed to injury risks abroad, travelers can advocate for injury control initiatives that might make the world safer for travelers and local populations alike. Therefore, potentially useful advice for the returning traveler and the travel medicine provider regarding injury control advocacy is offered.

ROAD TRAFFIC INJURIES

Epidemiology

More than 1.2 million people are killed on the world's roads each year.[14] Road traffic crashes were the eighth leading cause of death in 2010; by 2030, they are expected to be the fifth.[15] However, for those 15 to 44 years of age, road traffic crashes are the leading cause of death.[1,16] Eighty percent of road traffic deaths occur in middle-income countries, where rapid urbanization and motorization is taking place.[15]

For each death, another 20 to 50 persons are injured, some of which suffer permanent disability.[14,17] Without momentous global action, by 2020, RTIs are forecasted to be the third largest global disease burden.[14]

Differences in Road Traffic Injuries Between High-income and Low- and Middle-income Countries

In addition to the large road traffic burden in LMICs compared with high-income countries (HICs), several notable epidemiologic differences exist. In HICs, the most common road user killed by a road traffic crash is a car occupant, making up nearly 60% of road traffic fatalities.[15] In contrast, most vehicle occupant deaths in LMICs are passengers of minibuses, trucks, and other public service vehicles.[18] Pedestrians make up 22% of road traffic deaths globally, ranging from 10% to 66% of national road fatalities.[15] In LMICs, almost 70% of road deaths are vulnerable road users (VRUs, ie, pedestrians, motorists of 2- or 3-wheeled vehicles, bicyclists), compared to 40% in HICs.[15] This differential risk has consequences not only for health but also for social inclusion of people who cannot afford vehicular transport.[19]

Road Safety in Low- and Middle-income Countries

Road safety depends on 5 factors: political support, funding, and effective policies; safe roads; safe vehicles; safe road users; and timely, effective postcrash care.[15] The World Health Organization Global Status Report on Road Safety 2013 described road safety using this framework.[15] Particularly informative differences are described.

Only 7% of the world's population, most of which are in HICs, is protected by a funded, comprehensive road safety strategy. Consequently, road infrastructure is lacking and less maintained in LMICs than HICs. Safety structures (eg, guardrails, shoulders, streetlights) are often not planned, placed, or maintained. Although vehicle standards may be improving in LMICs, many vehicles remain less crashworthy compared with those in HICs (ie, older vehicle age; minimum safety regulations for imported vehicles; lack of seatbelts, airbags, or crumple zones). Lights, windshield wipers, and tires are often not replaced when needed. Nearly all minibuses and trucks that carry passengers in LMICs are not engineered to minimize the risk of passenger injury during a crash.

Well-established strategies to prevent pedestrian RTIs are poorly implemented worldwide, particularly in LMICs.[15] Road safety priorities and urban design neglect VRUs or fail to consider different risks for vehicle occupants and VRUs.[20] Further, drivers often do not respect VRUs, and VRUs often do not respect or know road safety signals.[21]

Poor enforcement and road user noncompliance limit the effectiveness of road safety policies. Only 26 of the world's 196 countries (13%) reported good speeding enforcement (8 or above on a scale from 0 to 10). Motorcyclist and/or bicyclist helmet use is poorly enforced by two-thirds of countries. Helmet standards are rarely incorporated into helmet laws. Drunk-driving laws do not protect 34% of the world's population. In Accra, Ghana's capital, 21% of randomly selected drivers had a blood alcohol concentration higher than 80 mg/dL.[22] This is markedly higher than was found in similar studies from Denmark (0.4%) and France (3.4%).[23] Additionally, 4% of bus drivers and 8% of truck drivers in Accra had blood alcohol concentrations of ≥80 mg/dL.[22] Seatbelts, child restraints, and mobile phone use while driving laws are particularly lacking or underenforced in LMICs.

Most RTI victims in LMICs do not have access to prehospital care. Good Samaritans and commercial drivers are the de facto ambulances in LMICs.[24] Resultantly, around 80% of injured patients in LMICs die before reaching a hospital, even in urban centers, compared with 21% in Seattle, Washington.[25] Hospitals often have critical deficiencies in resources necessary to provide essential trauma care.[3] Further, less than 55% of emergency care providers in Africa and Southeast Asia have had specific trauma care training.[15] Resultantly, injury for injury, victims in LMICs are at greater risk of death and disability than victims in HICs.[25]

Road Traffic Injury Risk Among Travelers

Travelers to LMICs are at twice the risk of RTI than their counterparts at home and more vulnerable than local populations.[8,9] In Bermuda, travelers were nearly 6 times more likely to sustain a motorcycle injury than Bermudians.[26] A regional hospital in Greece reported that only 15% of injuries were caused by road traffic among Greeks; among travelers to Greece, 40% of injuries were road traffic related.[27]

The effect of driving on different sides of the road on RTI risk is poorly understood. Studies suggest that travelers from countries that drive on the opposite side of the road than the country they traveled to are more likely to be injured than those that drive on the same side of the road.[27,28] RTI risk is not unique to tourists; business travelers are at higher risk as well. World Bank Group employees reported 1 road traffic crash per 175 trips.[29]

Pretravel Advice on Road Traffic Injuries

Despite these risks, much can be done to prevent RTIs in LMICs (**Table 1**).[30] Most of the recommendations should be practiced no matter the location; some are particularly important and are described here.

Table 1
Road traffic injury risks and recommendations to avoid them for travelers from high-income countries going to low- and middle-income countries

Risk	Recommendations to Avoid Risk
Lack of seatbelts, child safety seats, and airbags	• Select vehicles with seatbelts and wear them • If traveling with children, bring a child safety seat or booster seat • Ride as a backseat passenger when able • Rent vehicles with airbags if given the option
Travel when visibility or traction is limited or particularly dangerous, compounded by infrequent maintenance on vehicle components (eg, lights, brakes, windshield wipers)	• Avoid traveling at night or in the fog, rain, or snow • Avoid riding on overcrowded and overweight vehicles (eg, minibuses, trucks), particularly in these conditions, as they have a difficult time avoiding sudden hazards
Lack of signage or signage in a foreign language	• Drive with vigilance and caution • Do not react aggressively to other drivers' errors • Learn common signage before travel to avoid injury, putting others at risk, or breaking laws
Operating or riding 2- or 3-wheeled vehicles is high risk, as is being a bicyclist Unavailability of helmets	• Avoid travel on 2- or 3-wheeled vehicles if at all possible • If planning to operate or ride a 2- or 3-wheeled vehicle or bicycle, bring a properly fitting and approved helmet
Alcohol use	• Do not drive after consuming alcohol • Designate a driver before consuming alcohol
Being a pedestrian	• Take particular caution when crossing roads and look both ways no matter the direction of traffic • Seek and use crosswalks if available when crossing streets • Avoid walking along the roadside, particularly during times of limited visibility (eg, fog, night) • If driving, be especially cognizant of pedestrians and the risk you pose to them
Lack of emergency care	• Know the emergency access telephone number for the area(s) being traveled • Have a means of communication should injury occur • Create an emergency plan before traveling at the destination

Seatbelts and child safety seats reduce serious RTIs by 40% to 70%.[31,32] All possible efforts should be made to ride in vehicles with seatbelts and use them. Riding as a backseat passenger is safer than riding in a front seat, particularly when the vehicle lacks airbags.[33] Child safety seats and booster seats are rarely available in LMICs.[15] Travelers should bring them if traveling with children.

Road crashes are nearly 3 times more common during rain, at night, or during national holidays.[34,35] Thus, travelers should be advised not to travel in a vehicle at night, especially on undivided high-speed interurban or rural roads or during conditions that limit visibility or traction (eg, fog, rain, snow). If travelers are planning to drive, they should familiarize themselves with local laws, rent a vehicle with seatbelts and airbags, and pay particular attention to local driving hazards, namely, driving on the opposite side of the road than accustomed. Signage might be different or in a foreign language; travelers should familiarize themselves with common signage at their destination before departure to avoid injury, putting others at risk, or breaking laws.

Motorcycles or mopeds should be avoided at all costs. This advice should be stressed to travelers planning motorcycle use without significant experience operating these vehicles at their home. If a traveler must ride a 2-wheeled vehicle, a helmet should be worn. Helmets reduce the risk of death among motorcyclists by 42% in HICs with developed health care systems; the impact of helmet use among crash victims that don't have access to timely and effective trauma care is unknown but likely much greater.[36] Helmets that meet international safety standards are often not available in LMICs. If 2-wheeled travel is planned, travelers should be instructed to bring their helmet with them and wear it.

Alcohol use increases the risk of all causes of injury, particularly RTIs.[8] Travelers should not drive after consuming alcohol or ride with someone who has. Minibuses, trucks, and buses are often overcrowded, overweight and overspeed, which makes them prone to horrific crashes with high fatality and injury rates; thus, they should be avoided.[37]

Lastly, travelers will likely be pedestrians during their trip. Pedestrians should take particular caution when crossing roads and look both ways beforehand, paying particular attention to the side of the road drivers use; cross-walks should be sought and used when crossing streets if available. Walking roadside should be discouraged, particularly at night. Travelers planning to drive should be cognizant of VRUs and the risk they pose to them.

The effect of pretravel injury prevention advice on RTIs has not been studied. However, these simple risk avoidance recommendations are likely to reduce RTIs among this high-risk group.

DROWNING

Epidemiology

Around 350,000 deaths and more than 20 million disability-adjusted life-years are incurred from drowning annually.[16] Ninety-seven percent of this burden occurs in LMICs.[38] Drowning affects predominately young children in most regions regardless of national income.[16,38]

Drowning Risk Among Travelers

Drowning is responsible for 25% of injury deaths among US travelers and is the leading cause of death among travelers to Fiji, The Bahamas, Jamaica, Costa Rica, and other areas where water recreation is a major activity.[5,7] As with RTIs, travelers are 3 times more likely to drown abroad than they are at home.[9]

The greatest risk factor for child drowning in HICs and LMICs is a lack of supervision.[39] In LMICs, lack of supervision is complex and related to caring for several children, poverty, and increased maternal age.[40] Among travelers, lack of supervision is related to inattention to potential water hazards, distractions, and insufficient planning.[38] Other risk factors for LMIC populations include travel on unsafe or overcrowded watercraft and use of small boats for subsistence fishing.[41] Among travelers, unfamiliarity with local water conditions, alcohol use, and inability to swim are significant factors.[42]

Pretravel Advice on Drowning

Drowning is highly preventable; should it occur, medical treatment has little effect on the outcome.[43] Therefore, primary prevention is particularly important.[38] Pretravel advice should focus on risk reduction specific to the travel destination and planned activities. Personal floatation device (PFD) use and pool, open water, and boat safety should be discussed. Important points are listed in **Table 2**.

OTHER UNINTENTIONAL CAUSES OF TRAVELER INJURY

Aviation crashes, falls, burns, and injuries from adventure activities cause traveler deaths each year.[5] Like other causes of unintentional injury, many of these can be prevented. Specific risks and ways to avoid them are given in **Table 3**.

OPPORTUNITY FOR ADVOCACY

The preceding part of this article is oriented toward the need to sensitize travelers to the significant injury risks they face while abroad and to offer advice on risk reduction behaviors. When returning, travelers have shared risks with local populations. Therefore, they can be important advocates for the promotion of safety for everyone, everywhere.

In LMICs, injury control initiatives are often considered low priority by policy makers who must choose between competing issues.[44] Injury control is often neglected by policy makers because it is underresourced, requires a stance to be taken against industry, and is often impeded by political giants (eg, alcohol industry, firearm lobby).[45] To remove some of these barriers, the social value of injury control must improve and policy makers must be educated on the significant return on investment provided by injury control initiatives.

To heighten social awareness and educate policymakers about the burden of injury and cost effectiveness of its control, many stakeholders need to be involved.[45] Potentially important stakeholders include individuals and groups of citizens, nongovernmental organizations; industry; and governments. However, any group that campaigns for injury control and can positively influence social or political opinion should be included in advocacy efforts.[45,46] Advocacy can include the use of local or mass media (eg, flyers, newspaper editorials, radio shows), social media, direct political lobbying, or community mobilization through coalition of interest groups.[45] Successful examples of advocacy groups that started from a single or small group of individuals that have had a positive impact on injury control include Stop for Kids, Mothers Against Drunk Driving, and the Brain Injury Association of America.[45,47,48] Examples that include LMIC populations are few despite the greater burden they face.

Travel medicine providers also have a unique opportunity to advocate for injury control. Their understanding of the evidence base and position in society give their voice particular weight.[49] Many examples of physician-led advocacy groups that caused a significant national or international improvement in injury control exist (eg, Physicians

Table 2
Drowning risks and recommendations to avoid them for travelers from high-income countries going to low- and middle-income countries

Risk	Recommendations to Avoid Risk

Lack of PFDs or lack of PFDs that meet safety standards and fit properly	• Bring appropriate PFD when planning water activities
	• PFDs should be worn by:
	  ○ All children under 13 years
	  ○ Anyone who cannot swim
	  ○ Those participating in towed activities (eg, water skiing)
	  ○ Operators and riders of personal watercraft
	  ○ Sail or kite boarders
	  ○ Those on a vessel that is <26 feet in length, including those under paddle power
	  ○ Other situations.[38]

Low prioritization of pool safety Absent pool depth markings Potentially missing drain covers	• Feet first entry for every body of water • Inspect pools and spas before relaxing
Lack of lifeguards Ability for children to access bodies of water unattended	• All children should be supervised at all times by an adult who has not consumed alcohol • Delegate adult child supervision before water activities • Stay in accommodations that have lifeguards and a climb-resistant fence with a self-closing and self-locking gate if a pool is present • Ensure that staff do not permit children to bodies of water
Unfamiliarity with local water conditions, poor swimming ability, absence of lifeguards, and presence of rip currents	• Discuss conditions with local swimmers • Use the buddy system
Alcohol use	Do not operate or ride in a watercraft, swim, or supervise children after consuming alcohol
Unregulated SCUBA diving	• SCUBA dive only if certified by an accepted international organization • Ensure good health before diving • Check and be familiar with the dive center's gear • Use a diver-down flag • Use the buddy system
Unfamiliarity with operating or riding in a watercraft	• Avoid potentially dangerous watercraft (eg, over-crowded boats, undersized for conditions) • Identify locations of PFDs and fire extinguishers before departing • Do not underestimate the importance of boat safety courses, navigation rules, and the potential for dangerous weather or water conditions
Lack of emergency care	• Travelers should be competent in cardiopulmonary resuscitation • Know the emergency access telephone number for the area(s) being traveled • Have a means of communication should injury occur • Have an emergency plan

Table 3
Other injury risks and recommendations to avoid them for travelers from high-income countries going to low- and middle-income countries

Topic	Risk	Recommendations to Avoid Risk
Aviation crash	Small aircraft; developing countries	• Fly only on scheduled flights • Avoid small aircraft, particularly at night or during inclement weather
Fall	• Infrastructure not fitted for elderly safety • Open gutters, lack of guardrails, uneven stair depths, unmarked ground hazards • Child curiosity and growing sense of independence • Alcohol use	• Consider bringing mobility aid (eg, hiking poles, cane, walker) • Maintain vigilance when walking, going up stairs, or when at height • Closely supervise children • Responsibly consume alcohol • Delegate child supervision before consuming alcohol
Burn	• Lack of building codes or code enforcement • Lack of fire alarms and extinguishers • Lack of emergency access telephone numbers and formal fire services	• Stay on lower levels of accommodations to make escape or rescue easier should a fire occur • Identify at least 2 escape routes from the accommodation • Stay in accommodations with smoke detectors, fire alarms, and sprinklers if possible • Bring smoke detector
Adventure activity	• Lack of regulation or safety standards • Lack of communication networks • Lack of prehospital and trauma care, particularly in remote areas	• Be mindful of significantly increased risk of injuries with these activities • Bring safety gear that meets international standards (eg, helmets, harnesses) • Know the emergency access telephone number for the area(s) being traveled • Have a means of communication should injury occur; have an emergency plan

for Human Rights, International Campaign to Ban Landmines and Doctors Against Handgun Injury).[50–53] Physician-led unintentional injury control campaigns are less publicized.

Key messages that travelers and travel medicine providers might share during advocacy efforts include (**Fig. 3**):

1. Ninety percent of the near 6 million injury deaths annually occur in developing countries; 1 in 5 of these deaths is a child.[1,54]
2. Two-thirds of injuries are preventable.[11,12]
3. Families of the injured are frequently forced into poverty because of medical costs or lost wages, placing them at higher injury risk and creating an injury-poverty cycle.[55–57]
4. Road injury alone costs the world more than 500 billion dollars annually; some countries lose more on injury than they spend on health care.[56,58]
5. Injury control is as cost effective as human immunodeficiency virus/AIDS treatment and vaccination.[59,60]

Advocacy is a way for travelers to make a difference in LMICs that lasts long after their trip and for travel medicine providers to contribute to patient and population health more broadly.

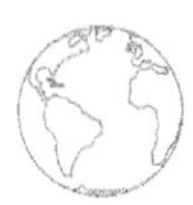

90% of the near 6 million injury deaths annually occur in developing countries; 1 in 5 of these deaths is a child.

Two-thirds of injuries are preventable.

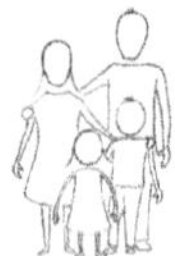

Families of the injured are frequently forced into poverty due to medical costs and lost wages, placing them at higher injury risk and creating an injury-poverty cycle.

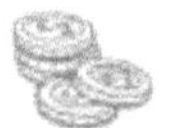

Road injury alone costs the world more than 500 billion dollars annually; some countries lose more on injury than they spend on healthcare.

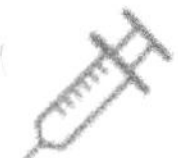

Injury control is as cost-effective as HIV/AIDS treatment and vaccination.

Fig. 3. Key points for injury control advocacy at home and abroad.

REFERENCES

1. Lozano R, Naghavi M, Foreman K, et al. Global and regional mortality from 235 causes of death for 20 age groups in 1990 and 2010: a systematic analysis for the Global Burden of Disease Study 2010. Lancet 2012;380(9859):2095–128.
2. Mock C, Juillard C, Joshipura M, et al. Strengthening care for the injured: success stories and lessons learned from around the world. Geneva (Switzerland): World Health Organization; 2010.
3. Wong EG, Gupta S, Deckelbaum DL, et al. Prioritizing injury care: a review of trauma capacity in low and middle-income countries. J Surg Res 2015;193(1):217–22.
4. Yeboah D, Mock C, Karikari P, et al. Minimizing preventable trauma deaths in a limited-resource setting: a test-case of a multidisciplinary panel review approach at the Komfo Anokye Teaching Hospital in Ghana. World J Surg 2014;38(7):1707–12.
5. Health information for international travel 2012. New York: Centers for Disease Control and Prevention; 2012.
6. Hargarten SW, Baker TD, Guptill K. Overseas fatalities of United States citizen travelers: an analysis of deaths related to international travel. Ann Emerg Med 1991;20(6):622–6.
7. Death of US citizens abroad by non-natural causes. Washington, DC: United States Department of State; 2014. Available at: http://travel.state.gov/content/travel/english/statistics/deaths.html. Accessed June 28, 2015.
8. Sanford C. Urban medicine: threats to health of travelers to developing world cities. J Travel Med 2004;11(5):313–27.
9. Tonellato DJ, Guse CE, Hargarten SW. Injury deaths of US citizens abroad: new data source, old travel problem. J Travel Med 2009;16(5):304–10.

10. Hill DR, Behrens RH. A survey of travel clinics throughout the world. J Travel Med 1996;3(1):46–51.
11. Wadhwaniya S, Hyder AA. Pre-travel consultation without injury prevention is incomplete. J Travel Med 2013;20(4):217–20.
12. Philippakis A, Hemenway D, Alexe DM, et al. A quantification of preventable unintentional childhood injury mortality in the United States. Inj Prev 2004;10(2):79–82.
13. Hanson DW, Finch CF, Allegrante JP, et al. Closing the gap between injury prevention research and community safety promotion practice: revisiting the public health model. Public Health Rep 2012;127(2):147–55.
14. Peden M. Global collaboration on road traffic injury prevention. Int J Inj Contr Saf Promot 2005;12(2):85–91.
15. Toroyan T, Iaych K, Peden M. Global status report on road safety: 2013. Geneva (Switzerland): World Health Organization: Department of Violence and Injury Prevention and Disability; 2013.
16. Data visualizations. Seattle (WA): Institute of Health Metrics and Evaluation; 2013. Available at: http://vizhub.healthdata.org/gbd-cause-patterns/. Accessed May 27, 2015.
17. Gosselin RA, Spiegel DA, Coughlin R, et al. Injuries: the neglected burden in developing countries. Bull World Health Organ 2009;87(4):246–246a.
18. Sethi D, Zwi A. Traffic accidents another disaster? Eur J Public Health 1999;9(1): 65–7.
19. Azetsop J. Social Justice Approach to Road Safety in Kenya: Addressing the Uneven Distribution of Road Traffic Injuries and Deaths across Population Groups. Public Health Ethics 2010;3(2):115–27.
20. Trevino-Siller S, Hijar M, Mora G. Prioritisation of road traffic injury interventions: results of a participative research with stakeholders in Mexico. Int J Inj Contr Saf Promot 2011;18(3):219–25.
21. Hijar M, Trostle J, Bronfman M. Pedestrian injuries in Mexico: a multi-method approach. Soc Sci Med 2003;57(11):2149–59.
22. Mock C, Asiamah G, Amegashie J. A random, roadside breathalyzer survey of alcohol impaired driving in Ghana. J Crash Prev Inj Control 2001;2(3): 193–202.
23. Ross HL. Prevalence of alcohol-impaired driving: an international comparison. Accid Anal Prev 1993;25(6):777–9.
24. Mock CN, Tiska M, Adu-Ampofo M, et al. Improvements in prehospital trauma care in an African country with no formal emergency medical services. J Trauma 2002;53(1):90–7.
25. Mock C, Jurkovich G, nii-Amon-Kotei D. Trauma mortality patterns in three nations at different economic levels: implications for global trauma system development. J Trauma 1998;44:804–14.
26. Carey MJ, Aitken ME. Motorbike injuries in Bermuda: a risk for tourists. Ann Emerg Med 1996;28(4):424–9.
27. Petridou E, Askitopoulou H, Vourvahakis D, et al. Epidemiology of road traffic accidents during pleasure travelling: the evidence from the Island of Crete. Accid Anal Prev 1997;29(5):687–93.
28. Page SJ, Meyer D. Tourist accidents. Ann Tourism Res 1996;23(1):666–90.
29. Goldoni Laestadius J, Selod AG, Ye J, et al. Can business road travel be safe? Experience of an international organization. J Travel Med 2011;18(2):73–9.
30. Mock C, Quansah R, Krishnan R, et al. Strengthening the prevention and care of injuries worldwide. Lancet 2004;363(9427):2172–9.

31. Final regulatory impact analysis amendment to Federal Motor vehicle safety standard 208. Washington, DC: Department of Transportation; National Highway Traffic Safety Administration; 1984. Contract No: Publication no. DOT-HS-806–572.
32. Kahane C. An evaluation of child passenger safety: the effectiveness and benefits of safety seats. Washington, DC: US Department of Transport; National Highway Traffic Safety Administration; 1986. Contract No.: DOT HS 806 890.
33. Smith KM, Cummings P. Passenger seating position and the risk of passenger death in traffic crashes: a matched cohort study. Inj Prev 2006;12(2):83–6.
34. Mogaka EO, Ng'ang'a Z, Oundo J, et al. Factors associated with severity of road traffic injuries, Thika, Kenya. Pan Afr Med J 2011;8:20.
35. Ngo AD, Rao C, Hoa NP, et al. Road traffic related mortality in Vietnam: evidence for policy from a national sample mortality surveillance system. BMC Public Health 2012;12:561.
36. Crandon IW, Harding HE, Cawich SO, et al. The impact of helmets on motorcycle head trauma at a tertiary hospital in Jamaica. BMC Res Notes 2009;2:172.
37. Odero W. Road traffic accidents in Kenya: an epidemiological appraisal. East Afr Med J 1995;72(5):299–305.
38. Cortes LM, Hargarten SW, Hennes HM. Recommendations for water safety and drowning prevention for travelers. J Travel Med 2006;13(1):21–34.
39. Hyder AA, Borse NN, Blum L, et al. Childhood drowning in low- and middle-income countries: Urgent need for intervention trials. J Paediatr Child Health 2008;44(4):221–7.
40. Ahmed MK, Rahman M, van Ginneken J. Epidemiology of child deaths due to drowning in Matlab, Bangladesh. Int J Epidemiol 1999;28(2):306–11.
41. Drowning. Geneva (Switzerland): World Health Organization; 2014. Contract No. Fact sheet N°347.
42. Gulliver P, Begg D. Usual water-related behaviour and 'near-drowning' incidents in young adults. Aust N Z J Public Health 2005;29(3):238–43.
43. Kyriacou DN, Arcinue EL, Peek C, et al. Effect of immediate resuscitation on children with submersion injury. Pediatrics 1994;94(2 Pt 1):137–42.
44. Debinski B, Clegg Smith K, Gielen A. Public opinion on motor vehicle-related injury prevention policies: a systematic review of a decade of research. Traffic Inj Prev 2014;15(3):243–51.
45. Sethi D, Mitis F. APOLLO policy briefing. Geneva (Switzerland): World Health Organization European Centre for Environment and Health; 2009.
46. Loue S. Community health advocacy. J Epidemiol Community Health 2006;60(6): 458–63.
47. Mothers Against Drunk Driving (MADD). Available at: http://www.madd.org. Accessed May 16, 2015.
48. Brain Injury Association of America. Available at: http://www.biausa.org. Accessed May 16, 2015.
49. Dharamsi S, Ho A, Spadafora SM, et al. The physician as health advocate: translating the quest for social responsibility into medical education and practice. Acad Med 2011;86(9):1108–13.
50. Hall P. Physicians for human rights (UK). BMJ 1991;303(6817):1562–3.
51. Kushner A, Raymond N. Health care hobbled: ambulatory care treatment of cambodian landmine survivors. J Ambul Care Management 2000;23(3):88–9.
52. Longjohn MM, Christoffel KK. Are medical societies developing a standard for gun injury prevention? Inj Prev 2004;10(3):169–73.

53. Kendrick D, Hayes M, Ward H, et al. Preventing unintentional injuries: what does NICE guidance mean for primary care? Br J Gen Pract 2012;62(595):62–3.
54. Harvey A, Towner E, Peden M, et al. Injury prevention and the attainment of child and adolescent health. Bull World Health Organ 2009;87(5):390–4.
55. Shrime MG, Dare AJ, Alkire BC, et al. Catastrophic expenditure to pay for surgery worldwide: a modelling study. Lancet Glob Health 2015;3(Suppl 2):S38–44.
56. Wesson HK, Boikhutso N, Bachani AM, et al. The cost of injury and trauma care in low- and middle-income countries: a review of economic evidence. Health Policy Plan 2014;29(6):795–808.
57. Thanh NX, Hang HM, Chuc NT, et al. Does "the injury poverty trap" exist? A longitudinal study in Bavi, Vietnam. Health Policy 2006;78(2–3):249–57.
58. Dalal K, Lin Z, Gifford M, et al. Economics of global burden of road traffic injuries and their relationship with health system variables. Int J Prev Med 2013;4(12):1442–50.
59. Bishai DM, Hyder AA. Modeling the cost effectiveness of injury interventions in lower and middle income countries: opportunities and challenges. Cost Eff Resour Alloc 2006;4:2.
60. Grimes CE, Henry JA, Maraka J, et al. Cost-effectiveness of surgery in low- and middle-income countries: a systematic review. World J Surg 2014;38(1):252–63.

Wilderness Medicine

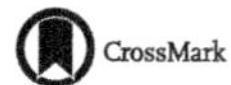

Whitney Alexander, MD[a], Steven Bright, MD[a], Patrick Burns, MD[a], David Townes, MD, MPH, DTM&H[b,*]

KEYWORDS

- Wilderness medicine • Preparation • Prevention and planning • Injury and illness
- Evacuation

KEY POINTS

- Traditionally, wilderness medicine encompasses prevention and treatment of illness and injury, education and training, emergency medical services, and search and rescue in the wilderness.
- As greater numbers of people pursue a wide variety of activities in austere, remote, and dangerous environments, wilderness medicine has evolved to include aspects of travel and tropical medicine, personal safety and security, and global and public health, in addition to its traditional components.
- Proper planning and preparation before venturing into the wilderness reduces the likelihood of injury or illness and helps mitigate the impact of injury or illness should they occur.
- Although injury and illness may both occur in the wilderness setting, traumatic injuries, including minor injuries, outnumber medical illness as the cause of morbidity in the wilderness.
- An important theme throughout wilderness medicine is to plan and prepare for the best-case and worst-case scenarios, and to be ready for the unexpected.

INTRODUCTION

Wilderness medicine is not easily defined, encompassing prevention and treatment of illness and injury, education and training, emergency medical services (EMS), and search and rescue (SAR) in the wilderness. Defining "wilderness" itself is challenging, as greater numbers of people pursue a wide variety of activities in austere, remote, and dangerous environments. In response, wilderness medicine has evolved to include aspects of travel and tropical medicine, personal safety and security, and global and public health, in addition to its traditional components.

[a] Division of Emergency Medicine, University of Washington School of Medicine, 1959 North East Pacific Street, PO Box 356123, Seattle, WA 98195, USA; [b] Division of Emergency Medicine, Department of Global Health, University of Washington School of Medicine, 1959 North East Pacific Street, PO Box 356123, Seattle, WA 98195, USA
* Corresponding author.
E-mail address: townesd@u.washington.edu

Med Clin N Am 100 (2016) 345–356
http://dx.doi.org/10.1016/j.mcna.2015.09.003 **medical.theclinics.com**

This inherent diversity of what constitutes the wilderness provides unique challenges for those charged with direct care provision, and wilderness medicine education and training of those venturing into these environments.

PLANNING AND PREPARATION

Proper planning and preparation before venturing into the wilderness reduces the likelihood of injury or illness and helps mitigate the impact of injury or illness should they occur.

Clothing

Proper clothing is essential for an enjoyable and, thus, successful journey into the wilderness. Clothing selection should focus on staying dry and warm, best achieved by layering garments that are waterproof/water resistant and breathable, provide insulation, and wick away moisture and dry rapidly.

Waterproof/water-resistant and breathable materials are ideal outer layers. These garments should be properly fitted and of high quality, as failure of this outer layer to keep one dry may result in an uncomfortable and potentially dangerous situation.

Beneath this outer layer should be insulating layers to maintain warmth. In wet environments this layer should contain materials that maintain their insulation properties even when wet. Such fabrics consist primarily of synthetic materials and some natural materials such as wool. In dry environments, down provides outstanding insulation and may offer some advantages over synthetics; however, down performs poorly if it becomes wet.

Materials that dry quickly and wick away moisture are best suited for the inner layer. Most of these are synthetic. Cotton, and similar materials that do not dry quickly and offer no insulation when wet, should be avoided.

Medical Kit

There are several considerations in deciding on the contents of a medical or fist-aid kit. The kit should be based on anticipation of need for the trip considering the location of the trip, the duration of the trip, and the number of individuals on the trip. The contents of the kit must not exceed the medical training, skills, and capabilities of the individuals on the trip. For instance, if there is no one on the trip with the proper training and experience to administer fluids intravenously, such fluids should not be included in the kit.

For each item in the kit, one should consider 3 characteristics: (1) the likelihood of use, (2) the potential impact, and (3) the cost that includes not only monetary, but size and weight. Emphasis should be on items that are likely to be used, have a significant impact on morbidity and mortality, and are inexpensive in terms of cost, size, and weight. For example, an epinephrine autoinjector is potentially life-saving if needed, and is relatively small and lightweight. Blister treatment materials are likely to be needed, reduce morbidity, and are inexpensive, small, and lightweight. If the trip includes travel to a developing country, antibiotics for traveler's diarrhea are likely to be used, reduce morbidity, and are relatively inexpensive, small, and lightweight.

Education and Training

In the United States there are various nationally recognized curriculum and education and training programs offering graduate-level wilderness medicine skills. The most basic of these is the Wilderness First Aid (WFA), which includes 16 hours of basic instruction in wilderness medicine. WFA is intended for the lay provider with little to no medical training or experience. Wilderness First Responder (WFR) offers a more advanced level of training. Courses generally run between 5 and 10 days depending on the schedule and content. Wilderness Emergency Medical Technician (W-EMT) courses combine formal EMT training with additional materials pertinent to the wilderness setting.

For health care providers there are professional organizations dedicated to wilderness medicine training and education. One example, the Wilderness Medical Society, offers advanced education and training opportunities through its journal published monthly, conferences held throughout the year, and programs including the Fellowship of the Academy of Wilderness Medicine.

PREVENTION

Waterborne Illness

In the wilderness, water may be contaminated with viruses, bacteria, or protozoa. Many can resist extremes of temperature and may survive in water for long periods of time. Common examples include *Giardia lamblia*, *Cryptosporidium*, *Shigella*, *Salmonella*, and hepatitis A virus.[1]

It is essential that all water collected in the wilderness be properly treated before it is consumed. There are several methods for treatment of water to make it potable. Ideally, 2 methods of water treatment should be available in the event one fails.

Boiling

Boiling water is a safe and effective method to kill infectious microbes. Most microbes are killed or inactivated at temperatures lower than boiling point; however, boiling is recommended because it is easy to recognize and does not require a thermometer. Recommendations that water is boiled for 3 to 5 minutes or longer at elevation are excessive and unnecessary, and waste fuel. Water must simply be brought to a full, rolling boil to be considered potable in terms of infectious microbes. Potential downsides to boiling water include the fuel required and the lack of removal of sediment.[1]

Halogens

Halogens, including chlorine and iodine, are generally easy to use and effective, and do not require the fuel needed for boiling. There are several disadvantages to using halogens. First, halogens do not neutralize *Cryptosporidium*. Infection with *Cryptosporidium* results in a self-limited diarrheal illness in immune-competent individuals but may be life-threatening in those who are immunosuppressed. Second, the ability of halogens to completely neutralize *Giardia* is unclear. Third, halogens, like boiling, do not reduce the sediment and, in the case of halogens, often leave the water with an unpleasant taste.[1]

Filtration

Filtration is probably the most commonly used method of water treatment in wilderness settings. In general, filters effectively remove sediment and larger enteric pathogens. The ability to remove smaller infectious agents such as virus and smaller bacteria depends on the specifications of the filter. Because viruses can be as small as 0.01 μm, an effective filter must contain very small pores. One disadvantage of filters with such small openings is that they take a long time to filter and are more likely to clog and stop working.

Ultraviolet radiation

Compared with the other methods, ultraviolet radiation (UVR) is a relatively new method of water purification. In sufficient doses, UVR will neutralize all enteric pathogens. Larger organisms, such as *Giardia* and *Cryptosporidium*, are particularly susceptible to UVR because of their large surface area. UVR works best in clear water without sediment.

There is no single best way to treat water in the wilderness, so a combination approach is often recommended. For example, water may be filtered to remove sediment and kill or inactivate large microbes, and then treated with a halogen or UVR to kill or inactivate smaller microbes. Similarly, water may be boiled to kill or inactivate microbes and then filtered to remove sediment.

Vector Control

In North America, insects, including mosquitoes and ticks, are primarily an unpleasant nuisance, but in some circumstances may transmit disease. There are strategies to decrease the number of insect bites including habitat avoidance, physical protection, and insect repellant.

Habitat avoidance requires a basic understanding of biting insect behavior. Mosquitoes and other biting insects are often most active at dusk; they prefer standing water and are attracted to light. Setting up camp away from standing water and minimizing artificial light will reduce the burden of biting insects.

Physical protection includes covering oneself with long sleeves and long pants tucked into socks. Tents and personal shelters may also provide physical protection against biting insects. Clothing and tents may be treated, or come pretreated, with permethrin, providing additional protection.

Insect repellants are another method of protection against biting insects. Generally considered most effective are those formulations that contain *N,N*-diethyltoluamide (DEET). Formulations range from 5% to 100% DEET. Concentrations greater than about 35% are unnecessary and offer little additional protection. In fact, the concentration of DEET has a greater impact on the reapplication time rather than overall protection. For example, 30% DEET offers no more protection than 20% DEET, but the lower-concentration product must be reapplied more often.

Picardin at 20% concentration offers an alternative to DEET with similar effectiveness, but is less caustic to synthetic materials and has a more pleasant smell.[1]

It is important to examine oneself daily for ticks. If a tick is found to have attached, it should be removed as soon as possible. Removal within 24 to 48 hours of attachment can significantly reduce the transmission of tick-related illness.[2]

There are many proposed methods to successfully remove a tick. Perhaps the most straightforward is to use a pair or blunt-end tweezers and grasp the tick close to the skin at its head and mouthparts, and provide slow and steady in-line traction. It is important not to use too much force or twist the tick, as this may leave the mouthparts attached to the skin. Application of caustic substances such as kerosene, alcohol, or a hot match is not recommended. Once the tick is detached, the bite site should be washed and monitored for signs of infection. Identification of the tick may help guide management should symptoms develop.

Sunscreen

Protection from solar radiation has important immediate and long-term advantages. Damage is primarily due to UVB radiation. The strength of sunscreen is expressed by its sun protection factor (SPF), which refers to the ability of a sunscreen to block UVB radiation only. UVA radiation has also been shown to cause skin damage, although the extent is less well studied.

There remains some controversy about which SPF is necessary. SPF greater than about 45 offers little additional protection. A sunscreen with SPF 15 blocks 93% of

UVB rays and a sunscreen with an SPF of 45 blocks about 98%. Regardless of the SPF chosen, all products must be reapplied if washed away while swimming, because of excessive sweating, if rubbed off, or if time has elapsed. In the most intense sun exposures, such as on high-altitude glaciers, it is reasonable to apply sunscreen every hour.

INJURY AND ILLNESS

Injury and illness may occur in the wilderness setting. In general, traumatic injuries, including minor injuries, outnumber medical illness as the cause of morbidity in the wilderness.[3] It is important to have basic understanding of the management of injury and illness, including being able to recognize or identify potentially serious injury and illness, and to provide definitive treatment of and initial management of minor injury and illness, stabilization, and evacuation of those patients with serious injury and illness.

When a situation with potential injury does occur, the first step is to assess situational or scene safety. This approach includes an assessment to determine whether the situation presents continued danger to those involved and those responding. One must consider whether the patient needs to be moved and whether it is safe for others to do so. Safety of both the patient and the responders must be considered.

In the initial evaluation of the ill or injured patient, one must assess the airway and breathing. Although other aspects of the patient's evaluation and treatment are important, airway and breathing should be assessed first. If the patient develops a problem with the airway at any time during the evaluation, it again needs to be the primary concern. It is not uncommon, especially for the inexperienced provider, to be distracted by more obvious injuries; however, it is important to keep the airway at the forefront of the evaluation. If the person is obtunded, the airway should be assessed and, if necessary, a jaw thrust or chin lift performed to improve or maintain the patency of the airway. Once the airway and breathing have been addressed, the evaluation should focus on circulation, deformity including any obvious injuries, and control of bleeding. If possible, significant bleeding should be addressed at the same time or immediately following airway and breathing.

Heat-Related Illness

Heat-related illness occurs when there is a failure of one's thermoregulatory mechanism, resulting in a net gain of heat from an inability to effectively transfer heat away from the body or from excess external heat gain. The spectrum of heat-related illnesses includes heat rash, heat cramps, heat syncope, heat exhaustion, and heat stroke.

Certain populations are at increased risk for heat-related illnesses, including the elderly and very young, as they are less effective at regulating body temperature. Patients taking medications, such as diuretics, β-blockers, antidepressants, and amphetamines, are also at increased risk as these medications can hinder the body's natural mechanisms to compensate in hot environments. Use of anticholinergic medications such as atropine, scopolamine, and diphenhydramine can increase the risk of heat illness by significantly diminishing the production of sweat.

It is possible to acclimatize to a warmer climate through progressive activity over a 1- to 2-week period. Sweat production will gradually increase at a lower skin temperature, resulting in more effective evaporative cooling.[4]

Prevention of heat-related illness begins with adequate hydration. As a general guideline, an individual should consume 0.5 to 1 L of liquid for every hour of strenuous activity. On a long wilderness trip, this requires having regular water sources or knowing when water will not be available and planning accordingly. Individuals should drink regardless of whether they feel thirsty, as thirst is not a reliable indicator of dehydration. Taking regular water breaks will help maintain hydration. Liquids that contain electrolytes, such as sports drinks, are preferred over water, because hyponatremia may develop if salt losses via sweat are not adequately replenished. Diuretics such as coffee, tea, and alcohol should be avoided.

Clothing that is lightweight, breathes easily, and worn in layers allows for improved temperature regulation. Dark-colored clothing will absorb heat and should be avoided in sunny environments.

Patients with minor heat-related illnesses such as heat rash, heat cramps, and heat syncope may be treated by relocating the patient to a cool, shaded area, having them rest, encouraging liquid intake, and gently stretching muscles that are cramping.

Heat exhaustion and heat stroke are life-threatening conditions. Patients with heat exhaustion may demonstrate headache, nausea, vomiting, dizziness, fatigue, and a rapid, weak pulse. Patients may progress to heat stroke, the hallmark of which is altered mental status that may include irritability, confusion, hallucinations, ataxia, seizures, or unresponsiveness. In both heat exhaustion and heat stroke the temperature may critically be elevated, typically around 40°C (104°F) or even higher. Although the core temperature is generally higher in heat stroke than in heat exhaustion, there is no specific cutoff discriminating between these 2 entities. Similarly, sweating should not be used to discriminate between these 2 conditions, as sweating may be present or absent in both heat exhaustion and heat stroke. Patients with heat exhaustion do not have altered mental status, whereas patients with heat stroke do.

The goal of therapy is rapid cooling to reduce the patient's body temperature. Patients with severe heat-related illness may lose the ability to autoregulate. The patient should be placed in the shade and have excessive clothing and equipment removed. If a vehicle is available, the patient may be placed in the vehicle with the air conditioning running. If the patient is alert, they should be allowed to drink cool liquids.

The patient may be immersed in cold water, although this is often impractical, and may result in too rapid a rate of cooling leading to shivering and unwanted heat generation.[5] A more practical method is to wet the patient's skin, preferably by misting with cool but not cold water, and fanning them to increase heat loss by evaporation. In addition, placing cold items, such as ice packs or cold water bottles, in the axilla and groin, and behind the neck will help cool the patient.

Antipyretics are not indicated for patients with heat-related illness. Dantrolene is not effective as a treatment for heat stroke.[6]

Patients with heat stroke are at high risk for morbidity and mortality, and should be evacuated.

Hypothermia

Hypothermia occurs when there is a reduction in body temperature secondary to excess heat loss or inability to generate heat. The severity of hypothermia is typically classified by core body temperature, as mild (35°–32°C), moderate (32°–28°C), and severe (<28°C). Patients with mild to moderate hypothermia demonstrate diminished fine motor skills, apathy, lethargy, and confusion. Shivering is the body's primary defense against hypothermia, and increases as body temperature approaches 32°C.[7] Shivering diminishes below a core temperature of approximately 32°C and stops below a core temperature of approximately 30°C, resulting in a rapid decline in core body temperature.

Patients with mild hypothermia may be rewarmed with passive rewarming, including removal from the cold environment, removal of wet clothing, putting on warm, dry clothes, and drinking warm liquids and eating carbohydrate-rich calories, allowing the individual to generate his or her own internal heat.

Patients with moderate and severe hypothermia will require active rewarming, which might include applying heat packs or warm water bottles to the axilla, chest, back, neck, and groin. It is important to use an insulating barrier layer to prevent thermal burns. Alternatively, if no heating source is available, body-to-body rewarming may be utilized if it does not result in a delay in evacuation. It is important to insulate the patient from the ground by placing insulating items such as a sleeping pad, a sleeping bag, or a tarp between the patient and the ground.

Patients who are severely hypothermic have decreased metabolic demands, and may show only minimal signs of life including shallow breathing, trace movements, or a slow and weak pulse. If they exhibit signs of life, cardiopulmonary resuscitation should not be initiated, as this may induce a fatal arrhythmia. These patients are susceptible to ventricular fibrillation, especially with rough manipulation, and therefore should be handled very gently. As it may be unrealistic to rewarm these patients in the wilderness, they should be maintained in a horizontal position, insulated to prevent further heat loss, and evacuated as soon as possible.

Allergic Reactions

Allergic reactions in the wilderness may occur after exposure to a wide variety of allergens including plants, insects, foods, or medications. Treatment includes preventing further exposure to the allergen by either removing the allergen or safely moving the patient.

Symptoms of a mild allergic reaction include hives, rhinorrhea, and watery eyes. Many of these are localized and self-limited. In addition to removal of the offending allergen, antihistamines such as diphenhydramine and ranitidine may alleviate symptoms.

Anaphylaxis is a life-threatening form of allergic reaction that can result in airway complications, gastrointestinal distress, and hypotension leading to anaphylactic shock. If the patient is has a swollen oropharynx, difficulty swallowing, change in voice, wheezing, shortness of breath, or signs of shock, epinephrine should be administered. In adults, the standard dosage is 0.3 mL of epinephrine with a concentration of 1:1000 administered intramuscularly in the lateral thigh. The standard pediatric dose is 0.01 mL/kg epinephrine with a concentration of 1:1000.

An epinephrine autoinjector is a common method of epinephrine administration for anaphylaxis in the wilderness. For the trained provider, ampoules of epinephrine, a syringe, and needle may also be used. Patients with a history of severe allergic reactions should carry epinephrine autoinjectors in the wilderness, and individuals traveling with them should receive instruction in their indications and use.

Patients who require epinephrine for anaphylaxis should be monitored closely, as they may require subsequent doses. Additional medications administered to these patients include corticosteroids such as prednisone, antihistamines such as diphenhydramine, and bronchodilators such as albuterol. It may be helpful to pack all of these medications together in a kit labeled "allergic reaction kit" for easy access in an emergency. In general, patients with anaphylaxis should be evacuated.

Head Injuries

In the wilderness it is often challenging to assess the severity of a head injury. The evaluation should include basic orientation questions to assess the level of consciousness, orientation, and recall of the event. If a person has undergone a fall with either immediate loss of consciousness or subsequent altered mental status, it should be assumed that, at minimum, they have mild cerebral concussion. Aspects of the patient's evaluation that should raise concern for intracranial injury include headache, vomiting, amnesia, ataxia, perseveration, and an inability to follow commands. Particularly high-risk patients include those who are intoxicated, the elderly, those taking anticoagulant medications, and those who have sustained multisystem trauma.[8] Though not intended for the wilderness setting, for some providers the Glasgow Coma Scale can be useful in initially assessing the level of consciousness of a traumatically injured person. It is important to have a high index of suspicion and to evacuate the patient if there is any concern for significant intracranial injury.

Spinal Injuries

Spinal injuries, especially of the cervical spine, are often a concern in patients with a suspected head injury. Patients with neck pain or tenderness, decreased level of consciousness, or neurologic symptoms should be considered to have a potential spine injury until proven otherwise. Although there are clinical decision rules for clearing a cervical spine in certain patients, including the Canadian C-Spine Rule and the NEXUS criteria, they should only be implemented by those adequately trained and experienced, and are not intended to be implemented in a nonhospital setting.[9,10]

If there is concern for cervical spine injury, the neck needs to be immobilized and the patient evacuated. In the wilderness setting, this often requires some improvisation with a malleable splint or rolled-up towels or clothing. During evacuation, care needs to be taken to maintain alignment and in-line stabilization of the spine.

Thoracic and Abdominal Injuries

Although some evidence suggests that thoracic and abdominal injuries are not common in the wilderness setting, because of their potential severity it is important to identify them and begin basic resuscitation if needed.[11] Thoracic and abdominal injuries may result from either blunt or penetrating trauma. Patients should be examined to look for bruising, abrasions, breaks in the skin, or other evidence of trauma.

Some blunt injuries, even significant ones such as rib fractures, pneumothorax, hemothorax, pulmonary contusion, and aortic injury, may have no obvious external signs of trauma.

Patients with pneumothorax and hemothorax will have decreased breath sounds on the affected side, and in the case of a tension pneumothorax the collapsed lung will be pulled toward the unaffected side, causing neck vein distension and tracheal deviation away from the side of injury; this may result in life-threatening hemodynamic instability if not decompressed. In the wilderness, needle decompression should be done only in the setting of hemodynamic instability.

Multiple rib fractures may result in a flail segment, whereby the chest wall moves paradoxically with respiration.

If penetrating trauma results in a large defect in the chest wall, the defect should be covered with a dressing that is sealed on 3 of the 4 sides. This chest seal allows air to escape on exhalation, reducing air entrapment and reducing the likelihood of developing tension pneumothorax.

Blunt trauma to the abdomen can cause a myriad of problems including injuries to the mesentery, bowel, spleen, liver, kidneys, and bladder. The spleen is the most commonly injured intra-abdominal organ in blunt trauma. Suspicion for these injuries should increase with certain mechanisms of injury, such as a fall from a significant height. The anatomic location of impact can help identify the most likely location of injury. If ecchymosis on the abdomen is present, with or without tenderness, this should further increase concern for a significant injury, and these patients require evacuation.[12] However, lack of external evidence of injury does not exclude the possibility of intra-abdominal injury. The presence of peritonitis, rebound tenderness, or a rigid or distended abdomen in the setting of blunt trauma indicates a significant injury, requiring evacuation.

Bladder injury should be suspected when there is an inability to urinate or gross hematuria in the setting of trauma. This situation requires immediate evacuation.

Patients with potential thoracic and abdominal injuries require evacuation. For penetrating trauma, a sterile dressing should be placed over the wound(s) before evacuation. Potentially serious thoracic and abdominal injuries are best managed in a hospital setting, and the goal of management in the wilderness setting is early recognition, basic management, and evacuation.

Musculoskeletal Injuries

Fractures and sprains

The most common type of injury in wilderness settings is musculoskeletal, including fractures, sprain, and strains.[3] Evaluation of an extremity injury should include the neurovascular status by palpation of distal pulses, assessing the temperature, and testing sensation. If the extremity is cool or pulseless, a significant vascular injury is suspected. When evaluating potential fractures, it is important to determine whether there is possibly an open fracture by looking for a break in the skin over the area of injury. If the extremity is angulated or deformed, it needs to be straightened and held in alignment or traction, especially if the deformity is associated with absent pulse. Once reduced or realigned, the neurovascular status of the extremity should be reevaluated. Traditionally traction has been preferred for femur fractures, although the data are unclear as to whether it provides an advantage over splinting.[13] Patients with open fractures, angulated fractures, suspected fracture-dislocations, or neurovascular compromise require evacuation.

Inversion and eversion injuries of the ankle resulting from hiking and climbing are common injuries in the wilderness. The Ottawa Ankle Rules provide a way to assess these injuries, and when performed by a properly trained individual help determine the need for ankle radiographs.[14] Under this algorithm, if the patient is unable to bear weight immediately or has tenderness at either the posterior aspect of the lateral or medial malleolus, there is an increased probability of ankle fracture. Although this approach does not definitively rule out a fracture and may be positive in a patient with a severely sprained ankle, it may have some utility in the wilderness setting.

Improvisation of splints for extremity injuries has long been part of wilderness medicine training; however, use of dedicated splints, such as commercially available malleable splints, is preferred. These splints are small, inexpensive, and lightweight, and can be used for many purposes including immobilization of both upper and lower extremities and the cervical spine.

Dislocations

Some joint dislocations that occur in the wilderness may be managed on site, whereas others require evacuation. Finger, patellar, and some shoulder dislocations, in particular, are potentially reducible in the field.

Finger dislocations most often occur at the proximal interphalangeal joint. With proper training, these may be reduced by applying traction to the affected digit while bringing the distal aspect of the digit up and over the proximal phalanx. Once reduced, the injured finger may be buddy taped to the adjacent digit for comfort.

In a patellar dislocation, the patella is displaced laterally. This dislocation may be reduced by slowly straightening the leg while pushing the patella medially.

The most common shoulder dislocations are anterior, with the humeral head anterior to the glenoid fossa. These patients generally should be evacuated, with the possible exception of those with previous shoulder dislocations who are able to reduce their own shoulder.

Wounds

Wounds encountered in the wilderness range from minor abrasions to complicated lacerations. The first principle of wound management is hemorrhage control. Often this can be accomplished with direct pressure for at least 15 minutes. If bleeding persists, evacuation should be considered. During evacuation, pressure dressings are the preferred method to achieve hemostasis.[15] Tourniquets should be reserved for trained providers for bleeding that is life-threatening or limb-threatening and does not respond to pressure. In these situations, tourniquets have been shown to decrease mortality with no increase in complications.[16]

The second principle of wound management, once hemostasis is achieved, is wound cleaning, best achieved by high-pressure irrigation with an adequate volume of fluid, namely at least 1 L for most small to medium-sized wounds. This aspect is especially important in the wilderness setting given the likelihood of a dirty wound. Sterile instruments and sterile irrigation fluid have not been shown to decrease rates of wound infection.[17] Water that is potable is generally sufficient for wound irrigation.[15]

Wound management in the wilderness will depend on the type of wound and the skill level and experience of the provider. Simple, small wounds not requiring closure may be dressed with a bandage or gauze and tape. Wounds requiring approximation of the skin edges may be closed with wound tape or Steri-Strips. Wound adhesive may be used in areas with low skin tension and wound edges that approximate easily. Sutures may be used to close wounds in the hands of a properly trained and experienced provider.

Complicated wounds, lacerations requiring multilayer closure, lacerations of the face, bite wounds, dirty wounds, and infected wounds should not be closed in the field.

Burns

Campfires and camp stoves are common causes of burns in the wilderness. Superficial burns are painful and erythematous, involving only the superficial layers of the skin. Partial-thickness burns involve part of the dermis, and present with blisters in addition to erythema. Blisters should not be unroofed in the field, as this could introduce infection. Full-thickness burns involve deeper tissues and can appear as leathery, white, or charred; they may be painless depending on the depth.

Superficial and partial-thickness burns may be treated with silver sulfadiazine or topical antibiotic ointment. Criteria for evacuation of burns patients depends on multiple factors including the depth and size of the burn, its anatomic location, adequacy of pain control, and potential for development of infection.

Blisters

Perhaps the most common and potentially avoidable injury encountered in the wilderness is friction blisters. These lesions commonly occur on the feet but may occur on the hands, especially when using hiking poles, or when cycling or paddling. A friction blister begins with a hot spot indicating irritation and inflammation of the skin. It is best to initiate treatment at this stage before a blister has formed, by placement of moleskin or similar commercially available material over the hot spot. In the absence of specific blister treatment, duct tape may be used.

If a friction blister has formed, the same materials may be used. Drainage of blisters is controversial except for those that look infected, which should be drained. Blisters that are drained or drain spontaneously should be cleaned, and a dressing or blister material applied. Similarly to other wounds, they should be monitored for signs of infection.

Prevention depends on wearing properly fitting shoe gear. Skin-toughening products are available over the counter, containing, for example, tincture of benzoin and isopropyl alcohol, and are marketed on the premise that applying them before a hiking trip may reduce the risk of blisters. These products seem safe and may help some individuals, although published evidence supporting their use is lacking.

EVACUATION

The decision to evacuate a patient may be difficult and complicated. Challenges include communication, logistics, and the implication of the evacuation on the remaining individuals. An additional challenge is determining whether the on-site individuals can or should evacuate the patient themselves, or require and wait for outside assistance.

Before venturing into the wilderness it is important to understand the options for SAR and evacuation, including how help is accessed (eg, mobile phone), how evacuations are performed, and who is financially responsible.

If the decision is made to wait for outside assistance, it is important to keep the patient warm and hydrated. Patients should be insulated from the ground and covered to keep them warm. Conductive heat loss by lying directly on the ground can lead to hypothermia. A sleeping pad, sleeping bag, extra clothing, or even brush or pine boughs may be used.

If the decision is made to evacuate a patient with on-site personnel rather than waiting for outside assistance, careful planning is essential, with special attention paid to how long it will take to reach help, which is often underestimated. If the evacuation will require staying in the wilderness overnight, it is important to bring the necessary supplies including water, food, shelter, and fuel.

In some situations where communication is unavailable, it may be necessary for someone to hike out to establish phone, radio, or direct communication with rescuers. Ideally, more than 1 individual should go for help while someone remains with the patient.

SUMMARY

Wilderness medicine combines planning and preparation, evaluation and treatment, education and training, and SAR in austere, remote, and dangerous environments. In addition to its traditional components, wilderness medicine has evolved to include aspects of travel and tropical medicine, personal safety and security, and global and public health. An important theme throughout wilderness medicine is to plan and prepare for the best-case and worst-case scenarios, and to be ready for the unexpected.

REFERENCES

1. Auerbach PS, editor. Wilderness medicine. 6th edition. Philadelphia: Elsevier; 2012. p. 877–1334.

2. Sood SK, Salzman MB, Johnson BJ, et al. Duration of tick attachment as a predictor of the risk of Lyme disease in an area in which Lyme disease is endemic. J Infect Dis 1997;175(4):996–9.
3. Montalvo R, Wingard DL, Bracker M, et al. Morbidity and mortality in the wilderness. West J Med 1998;168(4):248–54.
4. Cheung SS, McLellan TM. Heat acclimation, aerobic fitness, and hydration effects on tolerance during uncompensable heat stress. J Appl Physiol (1985) 1998;84(5):1731–9.
5. Smith JE. Cooling methods used in the treatment of exertional heat illness. Br J Sports Med 2005;39(8):503–7 [discussion: 507].
6. Bouchama A, Cafege A, Devol EB, et al. Ineffectiveness of dantrolene sodium in the treatment of heatstroke. Crit Care Med 1991;19(2):176–80.
7. Tikuisis P, Giesbrecht GG. Prediction of shivering heat production from core and mean skin temperatures. Eur J Appl Physiol Occup Physiol 1999;79(3):221–9.
8. Jagoda AS, Bazarian JJ, Bruns JJ Jr, et al. Clinical policy: neuroimaging and decision making in adult mild traumatic brain injury in the acute setting. Ann Emerg Med 2008;52(6):714–48.
9. Stiell IG, Wells GA, Vandemheen KL, et al. The Canadian C-spine rule for radiography in alert and stable trauma patients. JAMA 2001;286(15):1841–8.
10. Hoffman JR, Wolfson AB, Todd K, et al. Selective cervical spine radiography in blunt trauma: methodology of the National Emergency X-Radiography Utilization Study (NEXUS). Ann Emerg Med 1998;32(4):461–9.
11. Stephens BD, Diekema DS, Klein EJ, et al. Recreational injuries in Washington state national parks. Wilderness Environ Med 2005;16(4):192–7.
12. Hoff WS, Holevar M, Nagy KK, et al. Practice management guidelines for the evaluation of blunt abdominal trauma: the East practice management guidelines work group. J Trauma 2002;53(3):602–15.
13. Runcie H, Greene M. Femoral traction splints in mountain rescue prehospital care: to use or not to use? That is the question. Wilderness Environ Med 2015; 26(3):305–11.
14. Stiell IG, Greenberg GH, McKnight RD, et al. A study to develop clinical decision rules for use of radiography in acute ankle injuries. Ann Emerg Med 1992;21(4): 384–90.
15. Quinn RH, Wedmore I, Johnson EL, et al. Wilderness Medical Society practice guidelines for basic wound management in the austere environment: 2014 Update. Wilderness Environ Med 2014;25(4 Suppl):S118–33.
16. Beekley AC, Sebesta JA, Blackbourne LH, et al. 31st Combat Support Hospital Research Group. Prehospital tourniquet use in Operation Iraqi Freedom: effect on hemorrhage control and outcomes. J Trauma 2008;64:S28–37.
17. Valente JH, Forte RJ, Fruendlich JF, et al. Wound irrigation in children: saline solution or tap water? Ann Emerg Med 2003;41:609–16.

High-Altitude Medicine

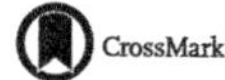

Nicholas J. Johnson, MD[a], Andrew M. Luks, MD[b,*]

KEYWORDS

- High altitude • Acute altitude illness • Acute mountain sickness
- High-altitude cerebral edema • High-altitude pulmonary edema • Prevention

KEY POINTS

- High altitude generally refers to elevations greater than 2000 m, although the risk of acute altitude illness does not increase significantly until individuals travel above 2500 m.
- Hypobaric hypoxia, the defining environmental feature of high altitude, leads to lower oxygen tensions at every point along the body's oxygen transport chain, which triggers multiple important physiologic responses.
- Travelers to high altitude should be prepared to prevent, recognize, and treat the 3 main forms of acute altitude illness: acute mountain sickness, high-altitude cerebral edema, and high-altitude pulmonary edema.
- The mainstay of prevention of acute altitude illness is gradual ascent; descent is the best treatment.
- Pretravel evaluation should include counseling about normal changes people experience at high altitude, the primary forms of acute altitude illness, and a systematic evaluation of the risks posed by any underlying medical conditions.

INTRODUCTION

Because of a growing interest in adventure travel, improved global travel infrastructure, and increased access to sites of historical and cultural significance, increasing numbers of people are traveling to high altitude. Although these individuals often enjoy amazing scenery and unperturbed landscapes, such travel is not without risk. All travelers ascending above 2500 m are susceptible to acute altitude illness, including acute mountain sickness (AMS), high-altitude cerebral edema (HACE), and high-altitude pulmonary edema (HAPE) while individuals with underlying medication conditions, even if

Funding: None.
Disclosures: The authors have no conflicts of interest, financial or otherwise, to report regarding the contents of this article.
[a] Critical Care Medicine, Division of Pulmonary and Critical Care Medicine, Harborview Medical Center, University of Washington, 325 Ninth Avenue, Box 359762, Seattle, WA 98104, USA; [b] Division of Pulmonary and Critical Care Medicine, Harborview Medical Center, University of Washington, 325 Ninth Avenue, Box 359762, Seattle, WA 98104, USA
* Corresponding author.
E-mail address: aluks@u.washington.edu

Med Clin N Am 100 (2016) 357–369
http://dx.doi.org/10.1016/j.mcna.2015.09.002 medical.theclinics.com

well compensated before travel, may be at increased risk for complications following ascent.

Given these risks, clinicians may encounter individuals planning high-altitude travel or who had problems on a recent trip. This article outlines a basic framework for counseling, evaluating, and managing these patients.

DEFINING "HIGH ALTITUDE"

Although no consensus definition exists, the term high altitude typically refers to elevations located above 2000 m (~6500 feet). Although observational studies have shown that individuals can develop acute altitude illness at elevations above 2000 m, the risk is not thought to increase substantially until individuals ascend above 2500 m (~8200 feet).[1,2] For most healthy individuals, it is only when traveling above this latter threshold that the altitude should be taken into account while planning a trip. For individuals with severe underlying medical conditions, such as severe chronic obstructive pulmonary disease (COPD) or pulmonary hypertension, the effect of the altitude may require consideration at lower elevations.

THE ENVIRONMENT AT HIGH ALTITUDE

With increasing altitude there is a nonlinear decrease in barometric pressure, which leads to decreased ambient partial pressure of oxygen (Po_2).[3] This process causes a decrease in the Po_2 at every point along the oxygen transport cascade from inspired air to the alveolar space, arterial blood, the tissues, and venous blood, which in turn triggers several important physiologic responses.

Other important environmental changes include increased ultraviolet light exposure, decreased humidity, and decreased ambient temperature, which increase susceptibility to sunburn and ultraviolet keratitis, dehydration, and hypothermia, respectively.

PHYSIOLOGIC RESPONSES TO HIGH ALTITUDE

Hypobaric hypoxia causes many physiologic responses across multiple organ systems, such as hypoxic pulmonary vasoconstriction, increased minute ventilation, and increased cardiac output (**Table 1**).[3] The magnitude of these responses varies between individuals, and this variability affects individual tolerance of hypobaric hypoxia and susceptibility to acute altitude illness.

As a result of some of these physiologic responses, travelers feel different at rest and with exertion at high altitude in comparison with lower elevations (**Box 1**). Reviewing these differences is a key component of pretravel counseling, as it can prevent misinterpretation of normal responses as evidence of illness and facilitate identification of individuals who are truly becoming ill.

ACUTE ALTITUDE ILLNESS

For most individuals, the risk of altitude illness begins with ascent to higher than 2500 m. Because health care providers may not be available for consultation during travel, all travelers should be able to recognize AMS, HACE, and HAPE, and respond appropriately if these conditions develop.

Acute Mountain Sickness and High-Altitude Cerebral Edema

Definitions and clinical features

AMS is a clinical syndrome characterized by headache plus one of several other symptoms including anorexia, nausea, dizziness, malaise, or sleep disturbance. It

Table 1
Physiologic responses to high altitude

System	Responses
Pulmonary responses	Arterial hypoxemia triggers increased peripheral chemoreceptor output leading to an increase in minute ventilation and a respiratory alkalosis Respiratory alkalosis blunts the initial ventilatory responses With continued time at high altitude, minute ventilation rises further because of renal compensation for the respiratory alkalosis and increased sensitivity of the peripheral chemoreceptors Alveolar hypoxia triggers hypoxic pulmonary vasoconstriction, leading to an increase in pulmonary vascular resistance and pulmonary artery pressure
Cardiac responses	Cardiac output increases, largely because of an increase in heart rate Stroke volume declines because of a decrease in plasma volume Myocardial contractility is preserved Systemic blood pressure increases to a variable extent
Renal responses	Variable increase in diuresis and natriuresis following ascent leads to a decrease in circulating plasma volume Arterial hypoxemia triggers increased secretion of erythropoietin (EPO) within 24–48 h of ascent Increased bicarbonate excretion as compensation for the acute respiratory alkalosis
Hematologic responses	Initial increase in hemoglobin concentration and hematocrit caused by reduction in plasma volume Over days to weeks, further increases in red blood cell mass, hemoglobin concentration, and hematocrit owing to increased EPO concentrations

typically occurs 6 to 12 hours following ascent above 2500 m, although the altitude at which symptoms start varies between individuals.[4] HACE is a severe, potentially fatal, form of altitude illness marked by signs of global neurologic dysfunction including truncal ataxia, altered mental status, and depressed consciousness. Although the underlying pathophysiology of these 2 disorders remains unclear, they are generally seen as being on the opposite ends of the spectrum of severity of a common process. Few individuals who develop AMS ever go on to develop HACE, but the onset of neurologic symptoms and signs in any AMS patient should always prompt concern for the possibility of HACE. AMS symptoms are not necessarily seen before the onset of HACE.

Box 1
How travelers feel differently at high altitude

Heart rate at rest and with any level of exertion is higher than at altitude of residence

Increased respiratory rate and tidal volume

More frequent sighs

Increased frequency of urination

Dyspnea on exertion that resolves quickly with rest

Difficulty sleeping including frequent arousals, insomnia, vivid dreams

Transient lightheadedness on rising to a standing position

Epidemiology and risk factors

AMS incidence is largely a function of the altitude attained and the rate of ascent, occurring in approximately 10% to 25% of unacclimatized persons ascending to 2500 m and 50% to 75% of individuals climbing Kilimanjaro (elevation 5895 m).[4–6] HACE is rare, having been reported to affect only 0.5% to 1.0% of persons traveling to 4000 to 5000 m,[4] although methodological issues make defining the true prevalence difficult. Although studies have sought to identify factors that affect risk such as age, gender, and weight, the most important risk factors for AMS and other forms of altitude illness remain the rate of ascent and prior history of altitude illness (**Table 2**).[4,5]

Prevention

The single best means to prevent altitude illness is to undertake a slow ascent to high elevation.[2,5,7] Above 3000 m, individuals should not increase the sleeping elevation by more than 500 m per day and should include rest days during which they sleep at the same elevation for multiple nights every 3 to 4 days. The altitude at which someone sleeps is considered more important than the altitude reached during waking hours.

A variety of medications are also available for prevention (see **Table 2**). Acetazolamide is the preferred agent, as multiple trials have demonstrated its efficacy in preventing AMS.[2,8,9] Dexamethasone is an alternative for individuals with intolerance of or an allergic reaction to acetazolamide.[2,9–11] Recent evidence suggests that ibuprofen may prevent AMS, but is not part of standard protocols at present.[2,12] Gingko biloba has also received attention in the research literature but is not recommended for this purpose.[2] Phosphodiesterase inhibitors have no role in AMS prevention.

Treatment

Descent is the best treatment for acute altitude illness but is not necessary in all circumstances. Patients with AMS should remain at their current altitude, and use nonopiate analgesics for headache and antiemetics for gastrointestinal symptom relief. Acetazolamide can be added to treat mild illness, while dexamethasone is very effective in the treatment of any severity of AMS, especially moderate to severe disease (see **Table 2**).[2,13,14] Individuals with AMS may ascend further once symptoms resolve, and should strongly consider continuing acetazolamide for the remainder of the ascent. Descent is indicated if symptoms fail to resolve after 2 to 3 days of appropriate treatment. Further ascent should never be undertaken in the face of ongoing symptoms.

Any individual thought to have HACE should descend to lower elevation. If descent is infeasible owing to logistical issues, supplemental oxygen or a portable hyperbaric chamber should be considered, if available (**Fig. 1**). Dexamethasone should also be started and no further ascent attempted until the individual is asymptomatic while off medications.[2]

High-Altitude Pulmonary Edema

Definition and clinical features

HAPE is a noncardiogenic pulmonary edema caused by exaggerated hypoxic pulmonary vasoconstriction and overly large increases in pulmonary artery pressure, which lead to leakage of fluid into the interstitial and alveolar spaces of the lung.[15,16] In the early stages, individuals have dyspnea beyond that expected for the level of exertion and altitude, loss of stamina, and dry cough. In later stages they manifest dyspnea with simple activities or at rest, cyanosis, and cough productive of pink, frothy sputum. HAPE typically develops 2 to 5 days after exposure to altitudes above 2500 m, but has

Table 2
Doses and other considerations for medications used in the prevention and treatment of acute altitude illness

Medication	Indication	Dose For Prevention	Dose For Treatment	Other Considerations
Acetazolamide	Prevention and treatment of AMS	125 or 250 mg every 12 h	250 mg every 12 h	Caution in renal failure; adjust dose for GFR[a] Contraindicated in patients with cirrhosis Avoid in patients with severe ventilatory limitation (FEV_1 <25% predicted) Caution in patients with documented sulfa allergy
Dexamethasone	Prevention and treatment of AMS and HACE	2 mg every 6 h or 4 mg every 12 h	AMS: 4 mg every 6 h HACE: 8 mg once then 4 mg every 6 h	May increase blood glucose values in diabetic patients Avoid in patients at risk for peptic ulcer disease
Nifedipine	Prevention and treatment of HAPE	30 mg sustained-release version every 12 h	30 mg sustained-release version every 12 h	Caution when combining with other antihypertensive medications
Tadalafil[b]	Prevention and treatment of HAPE	10 mg every 12 h	10 mg every 12 h	Avoid concurrent use of nitrates and α-blockers
Salmeterol[c]	Prevention of HAPE	125 μg inhaled every 12 h	Not used for treatment	Potential for adverse effects in patients with coronary artery disease prone to arrhythmia

Abbreviations: AMS, acute mountain sickness; FEV_1, forced expiratory volume in 1 second; GFR, glomerular filtration rate; HACE, high-altitude cerebral edema; HAPE, high-altitude pulmonary edema.

[a] Patients with a GFR of 10 to 50 mL/min should not take acetazolamide more frequently than every 12 hours; patients with GFR of less than 10 mL/min should not use the drug.

[b] Combination therapy involving calcium-channel blockers and phosphodiesterase inhibitors should be avoided.

[c] Salmeterol is not used as first-line monotherapy for HAPE prevention, and is generally reserved for use in addition to a pulmonary vasodilator medication.

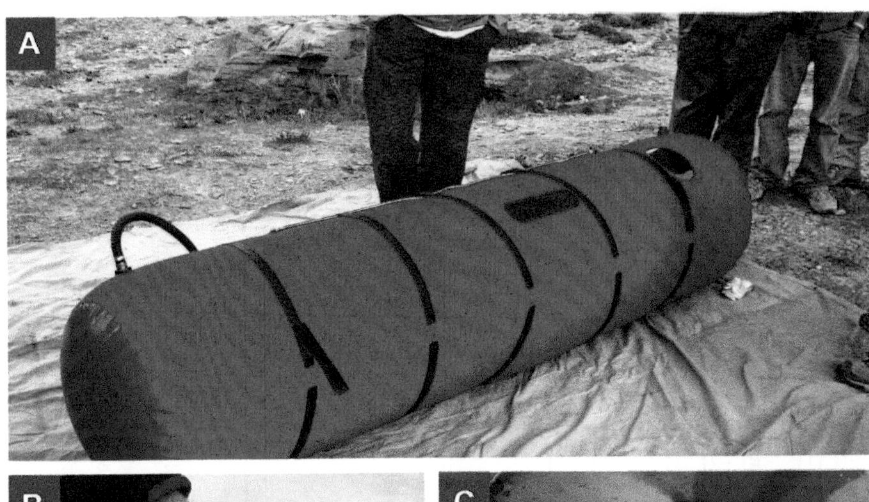

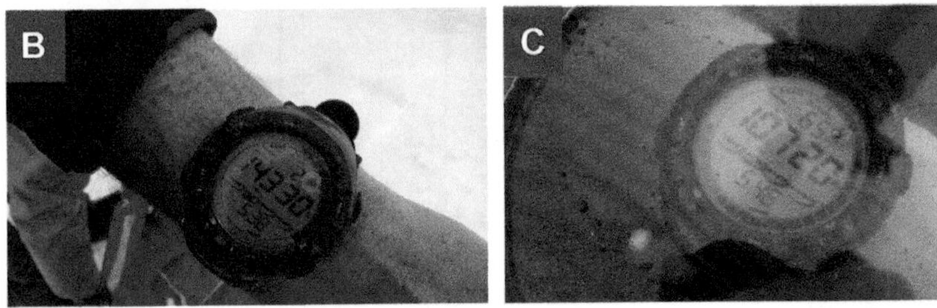

Fig. 1. Portable hyperbaric chamber. (*A*) Once an ill individual is placed inside the bag, a tight-fitting zipper is closed and the bag is inflated using a foot pump. Barometric pressure rises inside the bag, simulating a descent in altitude, as shown in the photo of an individual holding an altimeter watch outside (*B*) and inside (*C*) the bag following inflation. The magnitude of simulated descent varies based on the altitude of use and inflation pressure. Continuous pumping is required after initial inflation to maintain pressure and ensure adequate ventilation.

been documented at lower elevations in individuals with underlying pulmonary hypertension.[17]

Epidemiology and risk factors

The risk of HAPE is a function of the altitude attained, rate of ascent, and individual susceptibility. Individuals ascending to 4500 m have an incidence of 0.2% when ascending to 4500 m over 4 days, and an incidence of 6% when the same ascent is done within 1 to 2 days.[4,18] Studies from the Alps suggest that climbers with a prior history of HAPE have a roughly 60% chance of recurrence on future ascents to the same elevation at a similar rate.[4,18]

Prevention

Given the relationship between rate of ascent and incidence, gradual ascent is the best method for preventing HAPE. Extensive clinical experience, along with a small randomized trial, has established a role for nifedipine as the first-line agent for pharmacologic prophylaxis in individuals with a prior history of HAPE (see **Table 2**).[2,19] Dexamethasone, tadalafil, and salmeterol have also been shown to be effective in HAPE prevention in known susceptible individuals, but have not supplanted nifedipine for this purpose.[2,20] Acetazolamide can blunt hypoxic pulmonary vasoconstriction[21,22] but has not been shown to prevent HAPE, and should not be used for this purpose in known susceptible individuals.[7]

Treatment

If the affected individual can access a health facility, HAPE may be treated with rest and supplemental oxygen alone.[10,23] In the field, descent, supplemental oxygen, and nifedipine are the mainstays of therapy (see **Table 2**).[2,23,24] Care must be taken to avoid overexertion on descent, as this can raise pulmonary artery pressure and worsen HAPE. Phosphodiesterase inhibitors may be used as an alternative to nifedipine, although combination therapy should be avoided. If descent is infeasible because of logistical factors, supplemental oxygen or a portable hyperbaric chamber (see **Fig. 1**) should be used if available. There is no established role for acetazolamide, β-agonists, dexamethasone, or diuretics in HAPE treatment.

WHEN THE HIGH-ALTITUDE TRAVELER COMES TO CLINIC

Individuals may seek advice from their health care providers regarding high-altitude travel in 1 of 3 scenarios:

- *The altitude-naïve traveler* who has never ascended to high altitude before and seeks advice on how to ensure a safe trip.
- *The returning traveler* who had problems on a prior trip, and seeks information about what happened and how to prevent such problems in the future.
- *The potentially risky traveler* who has underlying medical problems that may worsen at high altitude or predispose to acute altitude illness.

The Altitude-Naïve Traveler

Many travelers have never been to high altitude, and seek advice about what to expect in this environment and how to prevent problems. Similarly, individuals who have traveled to high altitude before may be planning travel to a much higher elevation on a future trip, and seek advice about how their risk of problems may increase. These visits should include counseling about the normal changes to expect at altitude and the recognition, prevention, and management of altitude illness. A key decision is whether to prescribe pharmacologic prophylaxis against altitude illness. This decision should be based on assessment of the risk associated with the planned ascent (**Table 3**). Pharmacologic prophylaxis (see **Table 2**) is not indicated with low-risk ascent profiles but should be strongly considered for moderate-risk to high-risk ascent profiles.

The Returning Traveler

Travelers returning from high altitude often present for evaluation of problems that developed during their trip and how to prevent such issues in the future. A major challenge in these assessments is that the symptoms and signs have typically resolved by the time of evaluation, with little objective data available because travelers often do not access medical care at the time of their problem.

A key question is whether the problem was directly related to hypobaric hypoxia at high altitude. In general, symptoms and signs developing after ascent and resolving with descent are attributable to high altitude. The timing of onset relative to the ascent can also be useful, as AMS, HACE, and HAPE typically develop within 1 to 5 days of ascent and are extremely unlikely after 5 days at a given elevation.

Table 3
Risk categories for acute altitude illness in unacclimatized individuals

Risk Category	Description
Low	Individuals with no prior history of altitude illness and ascending to ≤2800 m Individuals taking ≥2 d to arrive at 2500–3000 m with subsequent increases in sleeping elevation <500 m/d and an extra day for acclimatization every 1000 m
Moderate	Individuals with prior history of AMS and ascending to 2500–2800 m in 1 d No history of AMS and ascending to >2800 m in 1 d All individuals ascending >500 m/d (increase in sleeping elevation) at altitudes >3000 m but with an extra day for acclimatization every 1000 m
High	Individuals with a history of AMS and ascending to >2800 m in 1 d All individuals with a prior history of HACE or HAPE All individuals ascending to >3500 m in 1 d All individuals ascending >500 m/d (increase in sleeping elevation) >3000 m without extra days for acclimatization Very rapid ascents (eg, Mount Kilimanjaro)

Abbreviations: AMS, acute mountain sickness; HACE, high-altitude cerebral edema; HAPE, high-altitude pulmonary edema.

Adapted from Luks AM, McIntosh SE, Grissom CK, et al. Wilderness Medical Society practice guidelines for the prevention and treatment of acute altitude illness: 2014 update. Wilderness Environ Med 2014;25:S7; with permission.

For individuals who developed acute altitude illness, prior performance at high altitude is a decent, but not perfect, predictor of outcomes on subsequent trips. Individuals with AMS and HACE do not warrant further testing to determine risk of recurrence, and can return to high altitude in the future. Because HAPE-susceptible individuals have a characteristic phenotype marked by excessive rises in pulmonary artery pressure in response to hypoxia and exercise, consideration can be given to evaluating for such responses in individuals with a concerning history, although this is not required in all circumstances. Whereas those with AMS may not require pharmacologic prophylaxis with future low-risk ascents (see **Table 3**), individuals with HACE or HAPE should use pharmacologic prophylaxis on future trips (see **Table 2**), as the consequences of these illnesses are potentially great. All individuals with prior altitude illness should receive counseling about the importance of slow ascent.

For problems other than acute altitude illness, the need for further evaluation depends on the particular problem. For example, individuals who developed chest pain on exertion at high altitude or those with symptomatic retinal hemorrhages may warrant further evaluation by the appropriate specialist.

The Potentially Risky Traveler

Although many travelers have no significant medical history, it is highly likely that some individuals who present for pretravel counseling will have underlying conditions that may pose a risk during the planned sojourn. These individuals warrant assessment to determine whether such issues will worsen at high altitude or affect the risk of acute altitude illness, particularly when the underlying disease is severe or affects the respiratory or cardiovascular systems.

A framework for assessing risk

Because information regarding the risks of travel with many of these problems is limited, providers can use a framework, based on 4 general questions, for determining the safety of the planned sojourn, the need for further pretravel evaluation, and the appropriate risk-mitigation strategies. Several issues related to specific medical conditions are addressed in **Table 4**.

Question 1: Is the individual at risk for severe hypoxemia or impaired tissue oxygen delivery? Although all individuals develop varying degrees of hypoxemia at high altitude based on the altitude attained and the strength of their ventilatory responses, certain categories of patients, including those with moderate to severe COPD, interstitial lung diseases, severe cystic fibrosis, and cyanotic congenital heart disease are at risk for severe hypoxemia and, as a result, increased dyspnea and poor exertional tolerance.[25,26] With anemia, the arterial Po_2 and oxygen saturation are the same at rest as in normal individuals but oxygen-carrying capacity and delivery are decreased, which may also lead to severe dyspnea and exercise limitation.

Question 2: Is the individual at risk for impaired ventilatory responses to hypoxia? Arterial hypoxemia normally triggers increased minute ventilation, whose role is to maintain alveolar and arterial oxygen tensions at adequate levels. Individuals with impaired respiratory mechanics, as in severe COPD, obesity hypoventilation syndrome, and many neuromuscular disorders, or those with impaired respiratory drives, such as following carotid artery surgery, may be unable to mount the expected ventilatory responses and, as a result, may be at risk for severe hypoxemia following ascent.[25]

Question 3: Is the individual at risk from the expected pulmonary vascular responses to hypobaric hypoxia? Decreases in the alveolar Po_2 following ascent cause hypoxic pulmonary vasoconstriction and an increase in pulmonary artery pressure. This change is well tolerated in most individuals but could pose problems for patients with pulmonary hypertension or right heart disease.[17,25,26]

Question 4: Will environmental features of high altitude or the expected physiologic responses to hypobaric hypoxia worsen the underlying medical condition? Certain features of the environment at high altitude or the expected physiologic responses to hypoxia can affect some medical conditions. For example, cold dry air may adversely affect airway function in asthmatic individuals,[27] while increased sympathetic nervous system activity can worsen blood pressure in hypertensive individuals. Hypoxemia at high altitude can trigger vaso-occlusive crises in patients with sickle cell disease or provoke myocardial ischemia in patients with poorly controlled coronary artery disease (see **Table 4**).[26,28]

Further evaluation

If the answer to all of these questions is "no," the individual is likely safe to travel to high altitude without further evaluation or risk-mitigation strategies beyond the general prevention measures described earlier.

For individuals deemed to be at risk based on nonreassuring answers to the first 3 questions, further risk assessment and risk-mitigation strategies may be necessary. One useful way to assess possible outcomes at high altitude is to expose patients to hypoxia and monitor their responses. The most feasible approach is the hypoxia altitude simulation test, whereby an individual breathes a hypoxic gas mixture while symptoms and physiologic responses are monitored.[29] The test can be supplemented with echocardiography to assess the pulmonary vascular responses to hypoxia. One challenge with the test is that its duration is short relative to the duration of the planned trip to high altitude, and may not reflect the full range of physiologic responses experienced by the patient during the trip. For individuals planning trips to distant places

Table 4
Common medical conditions and high-altitude travel

Disease	Key Issues For High Altitude Travel
Asthma	Well-controlled patients can travel as high as 6000 m. Data regarding travel to higher elevations are lacking, but such ascents are likely safe in well-controlled patients Avoid travel with worsening asthma control or following an acute exacerbation Continue inhaler regimen at high altitude and travel with an adequate supply of rescue medications. Keep inhalers warm in cold environments
Chronic obstructive pulmonary disease	Avoid high-altitude travel in patients with FEV_1 <1 L, CO_2 retention, pulmonary hypertension, or recent exacerbation Assess need for supplemental oxygen in patients with FEV_1 1.0–1.5 L Monitor pulse oximetry following ascent Continue inhaler regimen at high altitude and travel with an adequate supply of rescue medications. Keep inhalers warm in cold environments
Congestive heart failure	Avoid high-altitude travel with poorly compensated disease or following a recent exacerbation May ascend with well-compensated disease to altitudes <3000 m Monitor weight and blood pressure following ascent and adjust medications according to prearranged plan
Coronary artery disease	Avoid high-altitude travel with unstable angina, ischemia at low levels of exertion, or recent acute coronary syndrome (<3 mo, no revascularization) Consider risk stratification with stress test before travel Reduce level of exertion to slightly lower than that done at sea level Continue existing medications at high altitude
Diabetes mellitus	Increase frequency of blood glucose monitoring Avoid overly strict glucose control early in the trip because of concerns about glucometer accuracy a high altitude Evaluate for comorbid conditions (eg, coronary artery disease) that could worsen at high altitude Avoid vigorous exercise at high altitude if not experienced with high-level exercise at sea level
Hypertension	Mild or well-controlled disease: No indication for medication adjustments or routine blood pressure monitoring Poorly controlled or labile hypertension: monitor blood pressure following ascent and adjust medications for severely elevated blood pressures (>180/120 with symptoms or >220/140 without symptoms)
Obstructive sleep apnea	Patients with moderate to severe disease should travel with CPAP machine if access to power can be assured Consider adding acetazolamide to decrease the incidence of central sleep apnea
Pregnancy	Pretravel evaluation to ensure pregnancy remains low risk Avoid high-altitude travel with complicated or high-risk pregnancies (eg, impaired placental function, chronic hypertension, intrauterine growth retardation, anemia) Exercise at levels lower than at home; avoid dehydration Avoid travel to remote areas in the third trimester

(continued on next page)

Table 4 (*continued*)	
Disease	**Key Issues For High Altitude Travel**
Pulmonary hypertension	Avoid high-altitude travel without supplemental oxygen with moderate to severe disease (mean PA pressure >35 mm Hg or systolic PA pressure >60 mm Hg) In less severe disease, consider adding pulmonary vasodilator therapy or supplemental oxygen
Sickle cell diseases	Sickle cell anemia: avoid high-altitude travel because of increased risk of sickling and vaso-occlusive and splenic crises Sickle cell trait: high-altitude travel likely permissible, but patients should avoid heavy exertion and seek medical attention for left upper quadrant pain (possible splenic crisis)

Abbreviations: CPAP, continuous positive airway pressure; FEV_1, forced expiratory volume in 1 second; PA, pulmonary artery.

such as the Himalaya or Andes Mountains, another option, time permitting, would be taking test trips to mountain resorts or ski areas, where the individual can easily descend or access health facilities in the event of problems.

For nonreassuring answers to the fourth question, the approach varies according to the clinical circumstances. Further information about how to approach specific diseases is available in **Table 4** and in several reviews on these topics.[25,30–34]

SUMMARY

Travel to high altitude carries many rewards, but is not without risks. Travelers must be able to recognize, prevent, and treat the acute altitude illnesses and should receive pretravel evaluation for underlying medical conditions that may be affected by the altitude. Clinicians caring for such patients should be prepared to provide counseling about the normal changes at high altitude, stratify an individual's risk for altitude illness based on their planned ascent profile, and provide recommendations regarding prevention, recognition, and treatment of the main altitude illnesses and the management of underlying medical problems.

REFERENCES

1. Honigman B, Theis MK, Koziol-McLain J, et al. Acute mountain sickness in a general tourist population at moderate altitudes. Ann Intern Med 1993;118(8):587–92.
2. Luks AM, McIntosh SE, Grissom CK, et al. Wilderness Medical Society practice guidelines for the prevention and treatment of acute altitude illness: 2014 update. Wilderness Environ Med 2014;25(4 Suppl):S4–14.
3. Luks AM. Physiology in medicine: a physiologic approach to prevention and treatment of acute high altitude illnesses. J Appl Physiol 2014;118(5):509–19.
4. Bärtsch P, Swenson ER. Clinical practice: acute high-altitude illnesses. N Engl J Med 2013;368:2294–302.
5. Hackett PH, Rennie D, Levine HD. The incidence, importance, and prophylaxis of acute mountain sickness. Lancet 1976;2(7996):1149–55.
6. Karinen H, Peltonen J, Tikkanen H. Prevalence of acute mountain sickness among Finnish trekkers on Mount Kilimanjaro, Tanzania: an observational study. High Alt Med Biol 2008;9(4):301–6.

7. Bloch KE, Turk AJ, Maggiorini M, et al. Effect of ascent protocol on acute mountain sickness and success at Muztagh Ata, 7546 m. High Alt Med Biol 2009;10(1): 25–32.
8. Forwand SA, Landowne M, Follansbee JN, et al. Effect of acetazolamide on acute mountain sickness. N Engl J Med 1968;279(16):839–45.
9. Luks AM, Swenson ER. Medication and dosage considerations in the prophylaxis and treatment of high-altitude illness. Chest 2008;133:744–55.
10. Ellsworth AJ, Larson EB, Strickland D. A randomized trial of dexamethasone and acetazolamide for acute mountain sickness prophylaxis. Am J Med 1987;83(6): 1024–30.
11. Ellsworth AJ, Meyer EF, Larson EB. Acetazolamide or dexamethasone use versus placebo to prevent acute mountain sickness on Mount Rainier. West J Med 1991; 154(3):289–93.
12. Lipman GS, Kanaan NC, Holck PS, et al. Ibuprofen prevents altitude illness: a randomized controlled trial for prevention of altitude illness with nonsteroidal anti-inflammatories. Ann Emerg Med 2012;59(6):484–90.
13. Ferrazzini G, Maggiorini M, Kriemler S, et al. Successful treatment of acute mountain sickness with dexamethasone. Br Med J (Clin Res Ed) 1987;294(6584): 1380–2.
14. Levine BD, Yoshimura K, Kobayashi T, et al. Dexamethasone in the treatment of acute mountain sickness. N Engl J Med 1989;321(25):1707–13.
15. Swenson ER, Maggiorini M, Mongovin S, et al. Pathogenesis of high-altitude pulmonary edema: inflammation is not an etiologic factor. JAMA 2002;287(17): 2228–35.
16. Bärtsch P, Mairbäurl H, Maggiorini M, et al. Physiological aspects of high-altitude pulmonary edema. J Appl Physiol 2005;98(3):1101–10.
17. Luks AM. Can patients with pulmonary hypertension travel to high altitude? High Alt Med Biol 2009;10(3):215–9.
18. Bärtsch P, Maggiorini M, Mairbäurl H, et al. Pulmonary extravascular fluid accumulation in climbers. Lancet 2002;360(9332):571 [author reply: 571–2].
19. Bartsch P, Maggiorini M, Ritter M, et al. Prevention of high-altitude pulmonary edema by nifedipine. N Engl J Med 1991;325(18):1284–9.
20. Maggiorini M, Brunner-La Rocca H-P, Peth S, et al. Both tadalafil and dexamethasone may reduce the incidence of high-altitude pulmonary edema: a randomized trial. Ann Intern Med 2006;145(7):497–506.
21. Höhne C, Krebs MO, Seiferheld M, et al. Acetazolamide prevents hypoxic pulmonary vasoconstriction in conscious dogs. J Appl Physiol 2004;97(2):515–21.
22. Teppema LJ, Balanos GM, Steinback CD, et al. Effects of acetazolamide on ventilatory, cerebrovascular, and pulmonary vascular responses to hypoxia. Am J Respir Crit Care Med 2007;175(3):277–81.
23. Luks AM. Do we have a "best practice" for treating high altitude pulmonary edema? High Alt Med Biol 2008;9(2):111–4.
24. Oelz O, Noti C, Ritter M, et al. Nifedipine for high altitude pulmonary oedema. Lancet 1991;337(8740):556.
25. Luks AM, Swenson ER. Travel to high altitude with pre-existing lung disease. Eur Respir J 2007;29(4):770–92.
26. Luks A, Hackett P. High altitude and common medical conditions. In: Swenson E, Bartsch P, editors. High altitude: human adaptation to hypoxia. New York: Springer; 2014. p. 449–78.
27. Doan D, Luks AM. Wilderness and adventure travel with underlying asthma. Wilderness Environ Med 2014;25(2):231–40.

28. Bilo G, Villafuerte FC, Faini A, et al. Ambulatory blood pressure in untreated and treated hypertensive patients at high altitude: the high altitude cardiovascular research-andes study. Hypertension 2015;65(6):1266–72.
29. Dine CJ, Kreider ME. Hypoxia altitude simulation test. Chest 2008;133(4):1002–5.
30. Luks AM, Johnson RJ, Swenson ER. Chronic kidney disease at high altitude. J Am Soc Nephrol 2008;19(12):2262–71.
31. Bärtsch P, Gibbs JSR. Effect of altitude on the heart and the lungs. Circulation 2007;116(19):2191–202.
32. Luks AM, Swenson ER. Evaluating the risks of high altitude travel in chronic liver disease patients. High Alt Med Biol 2015;16(2):80–8.
33. Latshang TD, Bloch KE. How to treat patients with obstructive sleep apnea syndrome during an altitude sojourn. High Alt Med Biol 2011;12(4):303–7.
34. Richards P, Hillebrandt D. The practical aspects of insulin at high altitude. High Alt Med Biol 2013;14(3):197–204.

Adventure and Extreme Sports

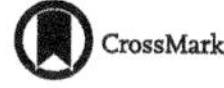

Andrew Thomas Gomez, MD[a], Ashwin Rao, MD[b,*]

KEYWORDS

• Adventure sports • Extreme sports • Adventure travel • Injury • Prevention • Skiing • Surfing

KEY POINTS

- Adventure and extreme sports include a variety of sports in varying environmental conditions, using specialized equipment.
- Injuries in these sports generally involve overuse, trauma, and environmental or microbial exposure.
- Understanding common injury patterns unique to each sport may aid in prevention and diagnosis.

INTRODUCTION

Adventure and extreme sports represent an array of physical activities that differ from traditional sports; they continue to attract a strong following. These sports, such as snowboarding, BASE jumping, and kayaking, involve a variety of unpredictable, often inhospitable environments, variable external conditions, high velocities, stunts, and specialized equipment. The increasing interest and participation in adventure and extreme sports, and the associated injuries, necessitates further understanding by clinicians.

This article aims to consolidate the findings of recent studies to aid clinicians in understanding, preventing, and treating injuries related to common adventure and extreme sports. These include alpine skiing and snowboarding, whitewater paddle sports, surfing, and bungee jumping. Two additional sports, BASE jumping and skateboarding, are also covered although travelers pursue them less often. Most of these activities offer varying degrees of physiologic challenge to the aerobic and

Disclosures: No conflicts of interest to disclose.

[a] Family Medicine, University of Washington, 331 Northeast Thornton Place, Box 358372, Seattle, WA 98125, USA; [b] Primary Care Sports Medicine Fellowship, Sports Medicine Section, Family Medicine, University of Washington, 3800 Montlake Boulevard, Box 354060, Seattle, WA 98195, USA
* Corresponding author.
E-mail address: ashwin@uw.edu

Med Clin N Am 100 (2016) 371–391
http://dx.doi.org/10.1016/j.mcna.2015.09.009 medical.theclinics.com
0025-7125/16/$ – see front matter

musculoskeletal systems, potentially reducing the risk of chronic medical conditions. Further research into these sports may offer insight into the relative risks and benefits to the participants' physical health.[1] During participation in these activities, injuries may result from overuse, trauma, or environmental or microbial exposure.[2]

ALPINE SNOWBOARDING AND SKIING

Overall Epidemiology

The National Ski Areas Association (NSAA) estimates that 44.7 serious injuries (paralysis, serious head injury, or other serious injury) occur among skiers and snowboarders each year.[3] Reassuringly, the NSAA commissioned 10-year studies, which started in 1980, and have found that injury rates have declined for both skiing and snowboarding.[4] The latest publication, with data from 2001 to 2010, indicated overall injury rates at 2.5 incidents/1000 visits for skiing and 6.1 incidents/1000 visits for snowboarding.[4]

Environment

According to the latest NSAA study, injuries to snowboarders more commonly occur on green (beginner) slopes compared with skiers (44.5% vs 40.6%), whereas skiers are commonly injured on blue (intermediate) slopes relative to snowboarders (51.6% vs 48.4%). There was no difference in injuries on black or double black (advanced, **Fig. 1**) slopes among skiers versus snowboarders. Most injuries occurred during on-hill activity (88% for skiing and 77% for snowboarding) as opposed to lift-related injuries (4.6% skiing and 4.1% snowboarding) or injuries related to terrain park use (4.9% skiing and 16.7% snowboarding) (**Table 1**). An increase in resort size is associated with lower incident rates.[4]

Demographics

Most participants are men and they sustain most injuries. Approximately 30% of participants on the slopes are snowboarders.[4]

Injury

Equipment and body mechanics differ between skiing and snowboarding, giving rise to varying risks and mechanisms of injury.[5] In general, most injuries in skiing and snowboarding occur as a result of impact with the snow.[4,6]

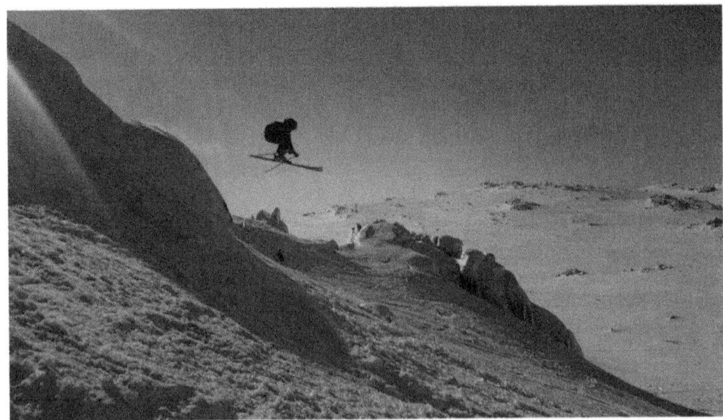

Fig. 1. Advanced, off-piste (nongroomed) skiing at Thredbo, New South Wales, Australia. (*Courtesy of* Robin Johnston (pictured), Whistler, British Columbia, Canada and Thredbo, New South Wales, Australia.)

Table 1
General mechanisms and environments of injury

General Mechanisms of Injury	Skiers (%)	Snowboarders (%)
On-piste (groomed trails) injuries	72	72
Terrain parks	19	25
Ski-lift related	6	3
Off-piste (nongroomed trails)	3	3
Falling down on same level	63	69
Loss of control related to jump	19	24
On-piste collision with another	8	3
Collision with static object	7	3

Data from Stenroos A, Handolin L. Incidence of recreational alpine skiing and snowboarding injuries: six years experience in the largest ski resort in Finland. Scand J Surg 2015;104(2):127–31.

Beginners are more likely to sustain an injury relative to those who are more advanced.[7,8] Among first-day participants, those younger than 17 years of age (odds ratio [OR], 3.16; 95% confidence interval [CI], 1.78–5.61) were at increased risk of injury relative to those in aged 26 to 40 years (OR, 1.96; 95% CI, 1.18–3.27).[9] In terms of general mechanisms of injury, beginners are more likely to sustain an isolated fall compared with more advanced snowboarders, whose injuries are related to high-impact forces, most often related to jumps.[6,7] In elite snowboarders, head injuries and wrist injuries decrease relative to the general snowboarding population, whereas shoulder, trunk, knee, and ankle injuries increase.[6] Jumping injuries occur more frequently in snowboarders (**Fig. 2**) relative to skiers (19.7% vs 15.7%), whereas skiers are 3 times more likely to collide with other participants compared with snowboarders.[3,4,6]

Relative to snowboarders, skiers are more likely to sustain lower extremity injuries caused by twisting or bending (15.1% vs 3.6%) as both legs can move independently.[4] Specifically, the knee is the most commonly injured anatomic site among skiers,

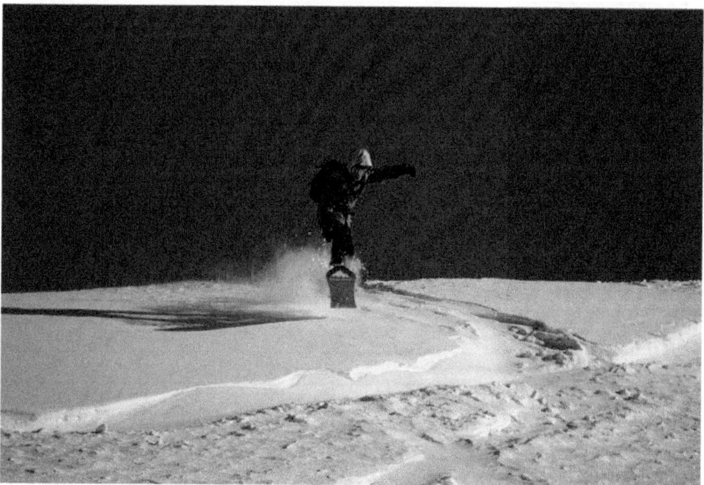

Fig. 2. Airborne snowboarder stabilizes himself with his left extremity in the air while landing a jump in La Parva, Chile. (*Courtesy of* Kevin McKenna (pictured), Beavercreek, OH.)

whereas the wrist is the most common site of injury for snowboarders. Some studies indicate that head injuries, including concussions, and fractures in general, are also more frequently sustained in snowboarders.[4–6] **Tables 2** and **3** further outline the anatomic regions and types of injuries. A variety of injury mechanisms in alpine sports that warrants further discussion includes ulnar collateral ligament (UCL) injury in skiers, upper extremity injuries in snowboarders, anterior cruciate ligament (ACL) injury, fracture of the lateral process of the talus (FLPT) in snowboarders, and spinal injuries.

Ulnar collateral ligament injury in skiers

UCL injury of the thumb commonly occurs among skiers who fall with an impact on an abducted thumb, specifically those who sustain a valgus force on an abducted thumb. A ski pole in the palm of the hand at the time of impact may act as a fulcrum. This injury commonly presents with pain, swelling, and hematoma along the ulnar border of the first metacarpophalangeal joint as well as pain and laxity on valgus stress testing. The diagnosis can be made clinically but MRI can confirm the diagnosis. Partial ruptures can be splinted with a thumb spica splint. Complete ruptures require surgical intervention.[10,11]

Upper extremity injuries in snowboarders

Upper extremity injuries in snowboarders commonly involve the wrist, upper arm, and elbow. Wrist injuries, as noted earlier, are the most common injury among snowboarders. In 1 study, wrist fractures occurred most frequently on the contralateral side relative to the leading leg (61.7%); shoulder dislocations followed a similar pattern (65.6%). Upper arm fractures (82.9%) and elbow dislocations (63.5%) occurred on the ipsilateral side of the leading leg. Wrist fractures (68.1%) and elbow dislocations (63.5%) occurred most often with backward falls, whereas shoulder dislocations (68.9%) and upper arm fractures (60.7%) occurred from forward falls.[12]

Anterior cruciate ligament injury

ACL rupture is a well-documented and well-described lower extremity injury among skiers; some of the most commonly described mechanisms include the following: boot-induced anterior drawer mechanism, “phantom-foot” mechanism,

Table 2
Anatomic regions of injury

Anatomic Regions of Injury	Skiers (%)	Snowboarders (%)
Head	16	16
Neck	2	2
Shoulder	11	12
Arm	4	10
Wrist	4	26
Hand	8	5
Thorax/abdomen	3	4
Back	6	9
Thigh	4	2
Knee	28	6
Lower leg	10	3
Ankle	5	6

Data from Ekeland A, Sulheim S, Rodven A. Injury rates and injury types in alpine skiing, telemarking, and snowboarding. Journal of ASTM International 2005;2(5).

Table 3
Types of injury

Types of Injury	Skiers (%)	Snowboarders (%)
Fracture	20	33
Dislocation	6	5
Sprain	26	20
Contusion	39	38
Laceration	8	5

Data from Ekeland A, Sulheim S, Rodven A. Injury rates and injury types in alpine skiing, telemarking, and snowboarding. Journal of ASTM International 2005;2(5).

valgus-external rotation, forceful quads muscle contraction, and the combination of internal rotation and extension.[13] ACL injuries in snowboarders occur when a snowboarder lands "flat" after a jump causing eccentric quadriceps contraction, loading the ACL. The ACL may be further strained when the knee is in valgus position on landing. ACL injuries are less common among snowboarders as the lower extremities are protected from rotational forces.[6,13] ACL injury management has been well documented and described.

Fracture of the lateral process of the talus in snowboarders

FLPT (known commonly as "snowboarder's fracture") is the second most common ankle fracture in snowboarders, after malleolar fractures, and accounts for 15% to 32% of ankle fractures in snowboarders.[13,14] This commonly misdiagnosed injury occurs as a result of dorsiflexion with ankle inversion combined with axial loading, specifically during high-impact injuries.[14] There are 3 types of FLPT: type 1 (avulsion), type 2 (large-fragment), and type 3 (comminuted). Less than 2 mm displacement can be managed with a short-leg cast and partial weight-bearing for 6 weeks. Large displacement fractures (type 2) should be managed by open reduction. Comminuted fractures should be treated to restore the anatomy.

Spinal injuries

Spinal injuries are reported to be more common among snowboarders relative to skiers (3.3% vs 1.4%). The thoracolumbar region is the most commonly affected region in both skiers and snowboarders; the most common type of fracture is an anterior compression fracture. Transverse process fractures more commonly occur among snowboarders[15] Spinal injuries occur as a result of falling in skiers, whereas failed jumps cause most spinal injuries in snowboarders.[16,17] Spinal cord injuries should be managed according to commonly accepted protocols.

Fatalities

According to the NSAA, in 2011 there were 5.5 fatalities per million participants; in the previous 10 years there were 41.5 total deaths per year on average.[3]

Prevention

All skiers and snowboarders should wear a helmet to prevent scalp lacerations and skull fractures, and reduce the severity of concussions.[4,7,18–22] Helmets have not been shown to increase cervical spine injury.[20,21] Snowboarders should wear wrist guards as they have been shown to decrease the risk of wrist injury, specifically sprains and fractures.[6,7,23] Educational materials or videos have been effective in reducing injury risk, collision, and falls in beginner skiers and snowboarders. One-hour educational workshops have been shown to be beneficial to more advanced participants. Skiers with injured knees can benefit from knee braces while skiing.[7]

SKATEBOARDING

Overall Epidemiology

There are currently 6 to 15 million skateboarders in the United States[24]; 66,000 to 85,000 injuries occur every year.[24,25]

National Electronic Surveillance System Injury data and exposure data from the National Sporting Goods Association indicated that 8.9 injuries occur per 1000 participants and 0.28 hospitalizations per 1000 participants.[26]

Environmental

Most injuries occur on public roads, skate parks, pedestrian walkways, and parking lots.[24,27] Other common locations of injury included residential areas, parks, and schools.[27] Many injuries occur as a result of an uneven surface or debris (rocks, sticks, ice).[24] Injuries requiring hospitalization were more likely to have occurred as a result of a collision with a motor vehicle (OR, 11.4; 95% CI, 7.5–17.5).[26]

Although skate parks create a dedicated and protected space for skateboarders, their creation has been associated with increased incidence of fractures and health care use.[24,28] Within the skate park, most injuries are associated with the use of ramps and rails (52.9%), followed by gullies (30.7%) and half-pipes (16.3%) (**Fig. 3**).[29]

Demographics

Most traumatic injuries among skateboarders involve teenage boys.[24,30,31] A 5-year study of data from the National Trauma Databank indicated that severe and critical injuries were more common among participants older than 16 years of age relative to those younger than 10 years of age, with a mean injury severity score of 8.6 ± 5.7.[31]

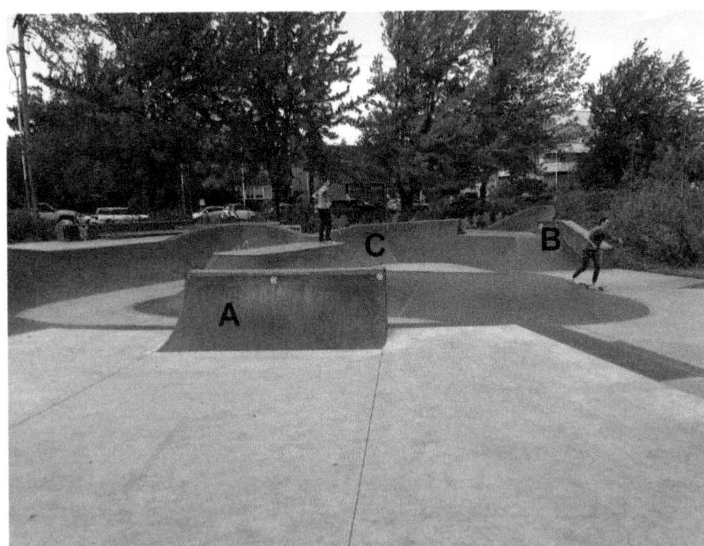

Fig. 3. Community skatepark in Northgate, Seattle. (*A*) a ramp, (*B*) a rail, and (*C*) a gully area.

Injury

Most injuries in skateboarding occur as a result of a multitude of factors, including intrinsic and extrinsic factors, rather than an isolated cause (for a discussion of external factors, see the Environmental section). Fatigue, overuse, and equipment problems all contribute to injury.[24]

The most common precipitants of injury include loss of balance or a failed trick.[27,30,32] Another documented cause of injury results from abruptly stopping on an irregular surface (described in the Environmental section), causing the skateboard to abruptly stop and the participant to lurch forward landing on a solid and unforgiving surface. Most skateboarders ride "regular" with the left foot forward as opposed to "goofy" with the right foot forward. Because most injuries occur on the left side, most injuries likely occur on the side of the leading foot or ipsilateral side of the leading foot.[24] Other documented mechanisms of injury involve a foot getting stuck between the board and riding surface, acute straining of limbs by one's own movement, being struck by an airborne skateboard during a trick, falling while riding downhill, and collisions with motor vehicles.[27,30,32] The remaining discussion on skateboarding injuries focuses on head injury, upper extremity injury, and lower extremity injury; see **Table 4** for anatomic distribution and types of injury.

Table 4
Anatomic locations of injury among skateboarders

Anatomic Location of Injury	Percentage
Head and neck	13.8
Intracranial	6.6
Fracture of neck, skull	0.6
Soft tissue injury	1.9
Sprain	0.1
Laceration	3.6
Dental	0.9
Upper extremity	50.9
Fracture	32.1
Soft tissue injury	12.0
Sprain	5.4
Laceration	1.3
Lower extremity	33.1
Fracture	11.9
Soft tissue injury	9.7
Sprain	10.1
Laceration	1.4
Trunk	2.1
Soft tissue injury	1.7
Sprain	0.4
Internal organs	0.2

Data from Keays G, Dumas A. Longboard and skateboard injuries. Injury 2014;45:1217.

Head injury

Among the cohort in the National Trauma Database, the overall incidence of traumatic brain injury (TBI), including concussion, severe TBI, and skull fractures was 36.3%, with increase of TBI associated with increasing age.[31] Other less severe head injuries include soft tissue injuries, lacerations, and dental injuries.[24]

Upper extremity injury

Upper extremity injuries account for more than half of all skateboarding injuries, making it the most commonly affected anatomic region, with the distal arm being most affected.[24,30,32] Injuries caused by falling on an outstretched hands (FOOSH) are common and involve significant impact forces with hard surfaces, ramps, rails, or stairs.[24,32] The upper extremity is also the most commonly fractured site (**Table 5**), frequently the result of FOOSH injuries, especially in older participants.[24,30] Fractures of the upper extremity were more common in participants 16 years of age or older relative to those 10 years of age or less.[24,31] Fractures of the ulna, radius, and wrist are the most commonly cited location followed by fractures of the clavicle and fingers.[30–32]

The most commonly fractured carpal bone is the scaphoid; identifying scaphoid fracture is crucial as avascular necrosis can result from decreased perfusion caused by displaced fragments.[24] FOOSH injury with the wrist dorsiflexed and radially deviated typically precipitates scaphoid fracture. The combination of swelling of the anatomic snuffbox, scaphoid tubercle tenderness, and pain with axial pressure on the first metacarpal bone has a sensitivity of approximately 100% for scaphoid fracture. Plain films and, if necessary, MRI can confirm the diagnosis.[33] Scaphoid fractures can be treated by a Colles cast or scaphoid cast not extending above the elbow for up to 12 weeks. Displaced fractures should be evaluated by an orthopedic surgeon.[34]

The elbow is often abraded during falls, but also commonly sustains contusions, sprains, and hyperextension injuries. "Skateboarder's elbow" results from a comminuted olecranon fracture causing loose bodies and long-term degenerative joint changes.[24]

Lower extremity injury

Injuries to the lower extremities commonly occur and include contusions, abrasions, lacerations, and fractures. Although knee injuries are infrequent relative to other locations, a variety of injuries can occur, including hyperextension, meniscal or chondral

Table 5
Skateboarding fractures treated at level I trauma center in Southern California in patients younger than 18 years

Fracture Location	Percentage
Forearm	48.2
Ankle	23.0
Elbow	12.6
Hand	5.8
Foot	4.2
Tibia	1.6
Clavicle	1.6
Humerus	1.0
Knee	2.1

Data from Zalavras C, Nikolopoulou G, Essin D, et al. Pediatric fractures during skateboarding, roller skating, and scooter riding. Am J Sports Med 2005;33:569.

lesions, and cruciate ligament injuries.[24] Participants younger than 10 years of age were more likely to sustain femoral fractures, whereas tibial fractures were more common in older participants.[31] Ankle fractures also commonly occur.[32]

Fatality

Only a few fatalities have been reported in the literature, most of which occurred when skateboarders collided with motor vehicles.[24]

Prevention

Helmets should be worn by all skateboarders as they may reduce the risk of injury and death.[24] A mouth guard may protect against dental injuries.[24,35] Elbow, wrist, and knee pads may protect against injury to the extremities.[24] Recommendations by physicians on personal protective equipment may improve compliance by providing easy access to helmets and other safety equipment.[36,37]

Other recommendations include safety instruction, formal training lessons, supervision, preactivity fitness and condition, and legislative efforts to promote the use of personal protective equipment.[24]

The American Academy of Pediatrics (AAP) has advised against the use of skateboards in children younger than 5 years of age because of limitations in neuromuscular development, higher center of gravity, and poor judgment. The AAP also recommends against participants riding in traffic and encourages communities to develop safe skateboard areas away from pedestrian and motor vehicle areas.[35]

SURFING

Overall Epidemiology

Surfing injuries occur at a rate of 2.7 to 4.0 per 1000 surfing days.[38] Among competitive surfers, 5.7 athletes are injured per 1000 heats.[39]

Demographics

Most injuries occur in men in their late 20s.[39–42]

Environment

Most acute injuries occur while riding waves during the summer months.[40,42,43] Larger waves, especially those taller than the participant, more than double the risk of injury relative to smaller waves (OR, 2.4; 95% CI, 1.5–3.9 and OR, 2.0; 95% CI, 1.3–3.3).[39,42] Surfing over a reef rather than a sandy sea floor also more than doubles the risk of injury (OR, 2.6; 95% CI, 1.3–5.2).[39] Tube riding or "getting tubed" (surfing inside a wave surrounded by water) is rare, yet accounts for a disproportionate amount of injuries.[39,42] Other injuries occurred while recovering the board, paddling, duck diving (diving under and through a wave), and entering or exiting the water.[39,42]

Injury

Nathanson and colleagues[39] found that most injuries occurred as a result of collision with one's own surfboard, particularly the fins. Contact with the sea floor was also a major cause of injury and was more common when surfing over a reef as opposed to a sandy sea floor. Most of the remaining injuries were caused by hydraulic forces followed by excessive and forceful body movements, primarily while carving during sharp turns. Injuries related to marine animals occur infrequently and often involve jellyfish, sea urchins, and stingrays.[42,43]

Most surfing injuries do not require inpatient management but risk factors for serious injuries include age greater than 40 years (OR, 1.9; 95% CI, 1.1–3.4), self-reported advanced surfers (OR, 1.6; 95% CI, 1.1–2.3), expert and professional surfers (OR, 1.9; 95% CI, 1.1–3.4).[39,40] Injuries requiring admission often include lower limb fractures, skull fractures, and cervical spine fractures.[40] Further discussion of injuries involves head injuries, ocular injury, otologic injury, extremity injuries, back injuries and surfer's myelopathy, dermatopathology, and chronic injuries.

Head injury

Most head and facial injuries occur as a result of superficial trauma and injury to this region commonly occurs (**Table 6**). However, a strike from a surfboard can cause skull and maxillofacial fractures.[38] Head trauma, whether from a surfboard or the sea floor, can cause concussion increasing the risk of near drowning.[42]

Ocular injury

Ocular injuries, including globe rupture and infraorbital floor fractures, often result when a part of the surfboard (fins, nose, tail) strikes the surfer.[38,44,45] An ophthalmologist should be consulted after eye trauma. Outcomes for these types of injuries are improving with advances in microscopy and vitrectomy enabling the salvage of eyes and restoration of vision that would have otherwise resulted in enucleation.[44] Prevention includes proper eye protection and covering sharper portions of the surfboard (fins, nose) with rubber.[38]

Otologic injury

Auditory canal exostoses are broad-based bony outgrowths that arise from the temporal bone and protrude into the auditory canal. The pathophysiology of these lesions is not well understood but prolonged and recurrent exposure to cold water (<15.5°C [60°F]) is a well-described risk factor.[38,43,46–49] Most are asymptomatic but may present with conductive hearing loss, chronic cerumen impaction, frequent ear infections and, occasionally, pain.[43,48] Barrier protection with earplugs may help prevent these lesions.[43,46]

Otitis externa may result from exposure to aquatic conditions, and causative organisms include *Pseudomonas*, *Staphylococcus aureus*, *Aspergillus*, and *Candida*. Treatment involves antimicrobial otic drops. Surfers should avoid the water for 7 days while being treated with otic preparations. Prevention may involve barrier protection with earplugs and/or the use of a 50:50 mix of acetic acid and isopropyl alcohol after surfing to facilitate drying of excess water in the ear canal.[38,43]

Tympanic membrane perforations result from water directly striking the ear, causing compression and rupture of the membrane. The pars tensa is most often involved, below the umbo and malleolus. Perforations often resolve without intervention, but

Table 6
Location of surfing injuries

Location of Injury	Percentage
Head/neck	36.6
Trunk	13.2
Upper extremity	12.6
Lower extremity	36.6
Systemic[a]	10.5

[a] Includes hypothermia and near drowning.
Data from Nathanson A, Haynes P, Galanis D. Surfing injuries. Am J Emerg Med 2002;20:158.

a repeat otoscopic evaluation should be performed within 2 weeks after injury. Auditory canals should be kept dry while the membrane heals. Tympanoplasty is reserved for severe cases.[38]

Extremity injury

The upper extremity is often injured with lacerations, shoulder dislocations, and hand injuries (finger fractures and dislocations).[42] Similarly, the lower extremity is commonly affected by lacerations followed by strains and contusions. Knee injuries often involve sprains and strains, meniscal tears, and dislocations often precipitated by rear foot slippage and forceful surfing maneuvers and carving.[38,42] Ample use of surfboard wax or deck traction can prevent foot slippage and routine warm-up and stretching may prevent injury.[38]

Back injury and surfer's myelopathy

Back spasms, resulting from isometric hyperextension of the spine during paddling, is the most common cause of disability among surfers.[38] Hyperextension of the lumbar spine has been implicated in spondylolysis and spondylolisthesis.[38,43] Additional thoracic injuries include rib fractures from impact with the surfboard and thoracic and spinal injuries related to sea floor contact.[38,50] Any surfer complaining of neck pain or who seems to be unconscious should be managed with appropriate spinal precautions, immobilization, and transport if necessary.[42]

Surfer's myelopathy is a relatively rare, nontraumatic spinal cord injury that occurs in novice surfers.[51] The injury occurs as a result of the surfer lying prone on the surfboard with the lumbar spine hyperextended for prolonged periods of time.[51,52] Other risk factors may include a thin, underdeveloped body habitus, weaker back musculature, dehydration, and possibly long distance travel.[52,53] Prodromal symptoms include back discomfort followed by variable motor symptoms, sensory symptoms, and/or urinary incontinence.[51,54,55] The cause is unknown but is likely ischemic.[51,52,56] MRI findings usually include a central T2-hyperintense signal abnormality in the spinal cord that often extends from the mid-thoracic region to the conus associated with cord expansion and varying degrees of conus enlargement; T1-weighted images are normal.[51,53,54] There is no established treatment and recovery varies from complete to persistent paraplegia.[51] Experienced surfers seem unaffected by surfer's myelopathy so swimming, surfboard paddling for endurance, strength training, and flexibility training may aid in prevention.[43]

Dermatopathology

Lacerations are the most common injury sustained and typically occur to the head, neck, face, and lower extremities resulting from impact with the sea floor or surfboard (see **Table 6**; **Table 7**).[38–40,42,43] Lower extremity lacerations most commonly occur from contact with hazards on the sea floor, including coral reef, rocks, and sea urchins.[38,42] Lacerations from coral reef contact are at risk of infection with *Vibrio*, *Alteromonas*, *Mycobacterium*, *Pseudomonas*, *Staphylococcus*, or *Streptococcus*.[38,43] Lacerations should be promptly irrigated, evaluated for retained foreign body, and treated on a case-by-case basis depending on severity and location. Topical or systemic antibiotics may be necessary in addition to tetanus prophylaxis.[43]

As well as lacerations, a variety of skin lesions commonly affect surfers, most of which are relatively benign. Sea ulcers result from untreated or undertreated lacerations, abrasions, or puncture wounds, most often affecting the distal extremities. Similarly, surfer's ulcers result from superficial erosions because of prolonged friction and pressure against the surfboard. These lesions occur on the lower anterior rib cage, tibial prominences, and the dorsal aspect of the feet. Surfer's dermatitis is a more

Table 7
Types of surfing injuries

Types of Injury	Percentage
Lacerations	42.3
Contusions	12.6
Sprain	12.0
Fracture	8.2
Concussion	5.9
Other[a]	19.1

[a] Includes abrasion, dislocation, bite/sting, tympanic membrane perforation, and tooth fracture/avulsion.

Data from Nathanson A, Haynes P, Galanis D. Surfing injuries. Am J Emerg Med 2002;20:158.

diffuse lesion caused by friction against the board combined with sunburn, sweat, and exposure to wind and surfboard wax. Other skin lesions noted among the surfing population include folliculitis (most often from *Staphylococcus aureus*), tinea versicolor, sunburn, and cold-induced angioedema. Surfer's sea ulcers should be kept clean and dry. Urea and balsam ointment, hydrogen peroxide, and isopropyl alcohol can provide further benefit. Recurrent ulcers may require debridement. Showering immediately after surfing and rinsing the wetsuit may limit outbreaks of skin infections. Sunburn may be prevented by adequate use of sunblock applied frequently and by use of wetsuits.[38]

Chronic injury

Chronic injuries result from overuse syndromes and environmental exposures. The most common overuse syndromes include shoulder injuries, back strain, neck, knee, and elbow strain.[43] Common upper extremity overuse injuries, related to the overhead nature of paddling, include shoulder impingement syndrome, acromioclavicular arthrosis, supraspinatus tendinitis, and other rotator cuff strains.[38,43] Treatment of these injuries has been documented, often among swimmers, and generally includes activity modification, physical therapy, rest and nonsteroidal anti-inflammatory drugs.[38,43]

Chronic marine environmental exposure predisposes surfers to external auditory canal exostoses (described earlier), and pterygium.[42]

Prevention

Surfers should be proficient at swimming and would benefit from an exercise and stretching regimen to reduce injury.[38] Surfers often do not perceive a need for personal protective equipment and use is further decreased by concerns about discomfort, claustrophobia, and alterations in vision, hearing, or balance.[38,57] Despite these concerns, surfers should be encouraged to wear helmets, eyewear, earplugs, and puncture-resistant shoes to reduce injury. Rubber pads placed on the surfboard nose and fins may further reduce the severity of injury during collisions with the surfboard.[38,42,43] Wetsuits may prevent hypothermia, and provide slight protection against abrasions and injuries related to marine animals.[38,43,57]

Surfing with a companion, avoiding hazardous surfing conditions, paying close attention to currents, water depths, and respecting warning signs may reduce the risk of injury. Awareness of the local flora and fauna may also assist in timely treatment of environmental exposures.[38]

BUNGEE JUMPING

Introduction

Injuries in bungee jumping are not well documented and limited to a variety of case reports, mostly involving injury to the eyes. Most injuries are related to the deceleration, often on the order of 2–3 *g*, but potentially upward of 8 *g*, occurring at maximal displacement.[58,59]

Injury

Case reports of ocular complications resulting from bungee jumping include retinal, macular, vitreous, and conjunctival hemorrhage.[58,60–66] Affected participants present with unilateral or bilateral blurry vision, scotoma, and decreased acuity.[58,60,62,63] Prompt intervention by an ophthalmologist may facilitate the restoration of normal vision.[58]

Other injuries related to bungee jumping include traumatic carotid artery dissection, pulmonary hemorrhage, left subdural hematoma, anterior dislocation of humeral head, comminuted proximal femoral fracture, peroneal nerve palsy resulting in foot drop, and quadriplegia.[59,67–72] One report documented the failure of the bungee resulting in free fall safely onto an air cushion.[73]

Prevention

Given the lack of cohort studies, counseling participants remains challenging. Those interested in bungee jumping should have a thorough health examination before participating. Those with vascular disease, ophthalmic issues, and reduced bone density may be at risk for injury.

BASE JUMPING

Introduction

The first fatal parachute jump from a fixed object took place from the Eiffel Tower in 1912 by a French tailor and parachuting pioneer, Franz Reichelt. One year later, the first successful jump took place from a static object in Washington, DC, by Stefan Banic, a Slovakian immigrant to the United States. The acronym B.A.S.E. (now referred to as BASE) was coined in 1981 by Carl Boenish, a filmmaker, to describe the static objects that parachutists would jump from: buildings, antennae, spans (bridge or arch), and earth formations (cliff or other natural earth formation).[74]

BASE jumping is banned at many potential jump sites but remains legal in many countries and many locations in the United States. The liability issues after an unsuccessful jump underlie its illegality in many places. No specific laws presently exist against BASE jumping but 2 felonies, trespassing and reckless endangerment, are usually used against unauthorized jumpers.[74]

BASE jumpers are allowed unlimited access, without special permits, to the 148 m (486 feet) Perrine Bridge on Highway 93 in Twin Falls Idaho. It is also permitted at the 267 m (876 feet) New River Gorge Bridge every third Sunday in October, known as "Bridge Day."[75] More formalized competitions take place at Kuala Lumpur's Petronas Towers, Colorado's Royal Gorge Bridge, and a variety of other venues around the world.[74]

BASE jumping participants often jump from heights of less than 152 m (500 feet) relative to the landing area, creating challenges in achieving aerodynamic stability given subterminal velocities.[74,76,77] BASE jumping uses a single canopy as opposed to a double canopy (like skydiving) and is associated with 5- to 8-fold risk of injury relative to skydiving.[74,75,77]

Overall Epidemiology

BASE jumping injuries occur in 0.2% to 0.4% of jumps.[76–78]

Demographics

Most injuries occur to single men in their 30s. Most participants have witnessed the death or serious injury of another BASE participant.[76]

Injury

The leading cause of serious injury and death in BASE jumping is an off-heading opening, wherein the single canopy chute faces the wrong direction on opening, causing collision with an object, often the location from which the participant jumped.[77] Most injuries are related to object strike and bad landings, which occur concomitantly in many cases.[74]

Exact injury characteristics are lacking for BASE jumping as it is a relatively new sport and not well studied. Most injuries involve the lower extremities, back and spine, chest wall, and the head.[76,77] Most injuries in 1 cohort caused a participant to be sidelined for an average of 4.5 months.[76]

Fatality

One study analyzing the deaths occurring from the Kjerag Massif cliff in Norway found the fatality rate to be 0.4 deaths per 1000 jumps.[78] Another analysis by Westman and colleagues[79] found that 1 fatality, on average, occurred per 60 participants per year (1.7%).

WHITEWATER PADDLE SPORTS

Demographics

Most studies evaluating injuries in whitewater sports were survey based; most respondents were men in their 30s.[80,81] One study specifically evaluating injuries in commercial whitewater rafters found an equal sex distribution.[82]

Epidemiology

Among recreational and competitive whitewater paddlers, injury occurrence was 4.5 per 1000 participant days and at a rate of 0.08 injuries per participant per year.[80,83] Whitewater rafting injuries occurred at a rate of 0.26 to 0.44 injuries per 1000 participants.[83,84]

Injury

Whitewater injuries can be classified into 4 main categories: (1) traumatic injuries related to striking an object (in or out of the watercraft), (2) traumatic stress related to positioning and hydraulic forces, (3) overuse injuries, and (4) submersion and environmental injuries.[81,84] Most studies evaluated injury patterns in kayakers and whitewater rafters and further discussion includes only these 2 sports. The remaining discussion on injuries focuses on acute kayaking injuries, acute rafting injuries, chronic injuries, and illnesses.

Acute kayak injuries

Blisters have been reported as the most common injury with most lesions occurring on the hands followed by the feet.[80,81] As well as blisters, which are most often benign, most injuries to kayakers occur either in the water after the participant has abandoned the kayak or while the participant is in the craft and is injured by hydraulic forces acting on the paddler's equipment.[81,83,84] Increased days spent kayaking per season and increased kayaker skill level were protective against injury in 1 study.[84]

Shoulder injuries, notably shoulder dislocations (5%–15% of all injuries), are common among kayakers.[80,81,84] The primary cause of shoulder dislocation involves improper or poor technique as paddlers abduct and externally rotate at the shoulder while paddling. Another risky maneuver that may precipitate shoulder dislocations is the "high brace," which involves using the paddle to prevent capsizing.[81]

Impact-related injuries most often involve the face, head, neck, and the lower extremities, and are likely related to collision with underwater hazards after submersion and swimming after capsize.[81,84] These injuries often involve lacerations, abrasions, and contusions. Closed head injuries are of particular concern given the risk of loss of consciousness and potential for drowning.[81,84] Novice kayakers sustain more impact-related injuries as a result of increased frequency of capsize.[83]

Acute rafting injuries

Rafters also face similar injury mechanisms to kayakers but different equipment leads to different injury risks. Most injuries occur while the participant is in the raft, often resulting from being struck by a paddle or other rafting equipment (**Fig. 4**), or related to being ejected from the raft and swimming in treacherous waters (**Fig. 5**).[81–83]

Most injuries sustained among rafters are minor and most often involve lacerations, followed by sprains, strains, fractures, contusions, and dislocations (**Table 8**).[82–84] The face (eye, mouth, nose, and teeth) and knee were the areas most often affected.[82,84] Other commonly affected regions include the extremities, torso, head, and neck.[82]

Injuries that occurred in the raft were more likely to occur to the face, whereas injuries sustained outside the raft, in the water, occurred commonly to the face and lower extremities. Women were more likely to sustain facial lacerations, whereas men were reported more likely to sustain injuries to extremities and torso in 1 study. This was likely the result of women having a tendency to sit in the middle or rear of the raft, assuming these positions to be less hazardous. Often, passengers from the front tend to be thrown backward, colliding with passengers in the middle and rear

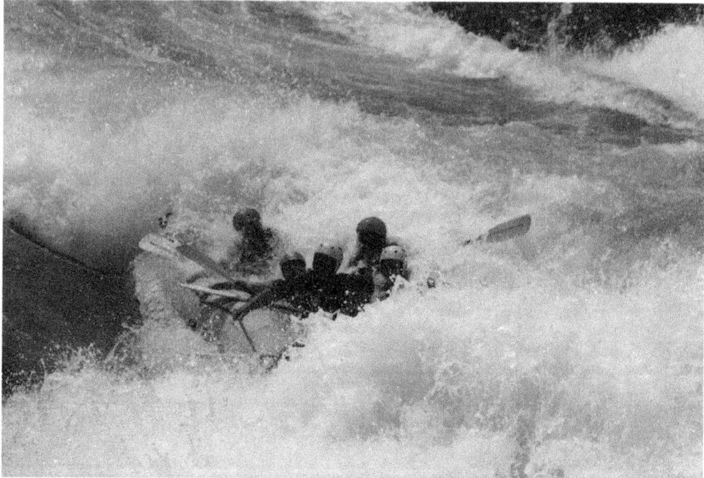

Fig. 4. Participants whitewater rafting in turbulent whitewater and at risk for injury-related collision with equipment inside the raft. Taken on the Nile near Jinja, Uganda. (*Courtesy of* Christopher Sanford, MD, MPH, DTM&H, Seattle, WA.)

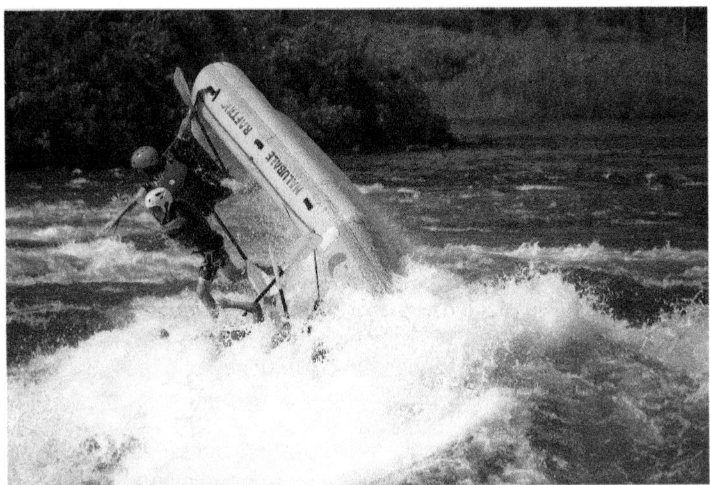

Fig. 5. Participants during raft capsize on the Nile near Jinja, Uganda. (*Courtesy of* Christopher Sanford, MD, MPH, DTM&H, Seattle, WA.)

of raft, potentially resulting in lacerations and other injuries. Furthermore, this association may be explained by men having a tendency to navigate riskier whitewater.[82]

Chronic injury

In general, chronic injuries manifest as tendinitis, sprains, and strains among kayakers.[80,83] The upper extremities are more often affected by overuse injuries, primarily involving the shoulder or wrist. The shoulder is vulnerable to overuse because of improper or poor technique, whereas the wrist is susceptible to DeQuervain tenosynoviitis related to constant wrist flexion and extension during paddling.[81,83] Clearly, more experienced kayakers may be at risk for overuse injuries.[84] A large fraction of whitewater rafters are infrequent commercial participants, and overuse and chronic injury data are lacking.[81] Among whitewater participants, injuries that resulted in the most time away from the sport (>24 months) included those to the back, shoulder, and wrist.[80]

Illnesses

Illnesses that occur in whitewater paddlers involve exposure to environmental and infectious dangers.[83] Leptospirosis is a zoonotic disease of worldwide distribution, but

Table 8
Types of injury among commercial whitewater rafters

Type of Injury	Percentage
Lacerations	32.5
Sprains/strains	23.2
Fractures	14.9
Contusions	9.8
Dislocations	8.2
Other	11.4

Data from Whisman SA, Hollenhorst SJ. Injuries in commercial whitewater rafting. Clin J Sport Med 1999;9:18–23.

endemic to the tropics, that causes an acute febrile illness.[84,85] Humans are infected through exposure to contaminated water or soil, often from infected animal urine, entering through abraded skin, mucous membranes, or conjunctiva.[85] Symptoms include fever, chills, myalgias, headache, vomiting, diarrhea, and skin rashes. Severe disease, known as Weil disease, may involve aseptic meningitis, jaundice, and renal and hepatic failure.[85,86] The Eco-Challenge-Sabah 2000 multisport endurance race held in Malaysian Borneo in 2000 involved kayaking as well as other endurance sports. Many participants during this race became infected with leptospirosis, and kayaking was the greatest risk factor for infection (relative risk, 3.3; 95% CI, 1.2–9.0) relative to other activities.[86] A similar outbreak occurred in Costa Rica among whitewater rafters.[85] Data suggest that chemoprophylaxis with doxycycline 200 mg weekly may be effective in the prevention of illness. Treatment of mild disease involves oral amoxicillin or tetracyclines, whereas more severe illness requires intravenous penicillin.[85,86]

Other reported illnesses or exposures include giardiasis, schistosomiasis, and hemlock poisoning.[80,84,87] One report documented a skin lesion infected with *Mycobacterium marinum* after a kayak injury.[88]

External auditory canal exostoses have also been reported, associated with prolonged and frequent cold water exposures, similar to surfers.[83,89]

Fatality

Fatalities have been documented in relation to 2 broad scenarios. The first involves inexperienced whitewater participants who get caught in situations beyond their capabilities, whereas the other involves experienced boaters, usually kayakers, attempting to navigate extremely dangerous whitewater.[81]

Fatalities have been documented as occurring in 2.9 whitewater paddlers per 100,000 participants per year in the United States.[83] Another study found an overall whitewater fatality rate of 0.87 deaths per 100,000 user days (kayakers, canoes, and private and commercial rafters).[90]

Prevention and Treatment

Most injuries incurred by whitewater participants are not obscure and require generally accepted techniques in identification and management. An appropriate health examination and risk assessment should be done before participating in whitewater sports. Expert advice should be sought about the specific river a participant plans to navigate. The correct equipment should be used.[83] Proper educational materials should be reviewed by participants.[91]

Personal protective equipment and flotation devices should be used at all times while paddling, including helmets, faceguard, and ear plugs. Ear plugs may prevent formation of external auditory canal exostoses.[89] Proper hygiene should be observed to prevent infectious illnesses.[83,91,92] Alcohol should be avoided.[91]

After paddling, the participant should have adequate rest to heal and recuperate. An effective training program may prevent injury.[83]

REFERENCES

1. Burr JF, Montelpare WJ, Shephard RJ. Do adventure sports have a role in health promotion? Need for objective evidence for a risk-benefit analysis. Can Fam Physician 2013;59:1311–3.
2. Young CC. Extreme sports: injuries and medical coverage. Curr Sports Med Rep 2002;1:306–11.

3. Hawks T. Facts about Skiing/Snowboarding Safety [Internet]. National Ski Areas Association; 2012 [cited 2015 Aug 5]; Available at: https://www.nsaa.org/media/68045/NSAA-Facts-About-Skiing-Snowboarding-Safety-10-1-12.pdf.
4. Shealy JE, Ettlinger CF, Scher I, et al. "2010/2011 NSAA 10-Year Interval Injury Study," Skiing Trauma and Safety: 20th Volume, STP 1582, Robert J. Johnson, Ed., pp. 93–111, http://dx.doi.org/10.1520/STP158220140002, ASTM International, West Conshohocken, PA 2015.
5. Stenroos A, Handolin L. Incidence of recreational alpine skiing and snowboarding injuries: six years experience in the largest ski resort in Finland. Scand J Surg 2015;104:127–31.
6. Wijdicks CA, Rosenbach BS, Flanagan TR, et al. Injuries in elite and recreational snowboarders. Br J Sports Med 2014;48:11–7.
7. Hume PA, Lorimer AV, Griffiths PC, et al. Recreational snow-sports injury risk factors and countermeasures: a meta-analysis review and haddon matrix evaluation. Sports Med 2015;45(8):1175–90.
8. Ekeland A, Sulheim S, Rodven A. Injury rates and injury types in alpine skiing, telemarking, and snowboarding. J ASTM Int 2005;2(5):31–9.
9. Langran M, Selvaraj S. Increased injury risk among first-day skiers, snowboarders, and skiboarders. Am J Sports Med 2004;32:96–103.
10. Ritting AW, Baldwin PC, Rodner CM. Ulnar collateral ligament injury of the thumb metacarpophalangeal joint. Clin J Sport Med 2010;20:106–12.
11. Anderson D. Skier's thumb. Aust Fam Physician 2010;39:575–7.
12. Yamauchi K, Wakahara K, Fukuta M, et al. Characteristics of upper extremity injuries sustained by falling during snowboarding: a study of 1918 cases. Am J Sports Med 2010;38:1468–74.
13. Mahmood B, Duggal N. Lower extremity injuries in snowboarders. Am J Orthop 2014;43:502–5.
14. McCrory P, Bladin C. Fractures of the lateral process of the talus: a clinical review. "Snowboarder's ankle". Clin J Sport Med 1996;6:124–8.
15. Yamakawa H, Murase S, Sakai H, et al. Spinal injuries in snowboarders: risk of jumping as an integral part of snowboarding. J Trauma 2001;50:1101–5.
16. Wakahara K, Matsumoto K, Sumi H, et al. Traumatic spinal cord injuries from snowboarding. Am J Sports Med 2006;34:1670–4.
17. Tarazi F, Dvorak MF, Wing PC. Spinal injuries in skiers and snowboarders. Am J Sports Med 1999;27:177–80.
18. Shealy JE., Johnson RJ., Ettlinger CF, et al. "Role of Helmets in Mitigation of Head Injuries: Epidemiologic Study of Head Injuries to Skiers," Skiing Trauma and Safety: 20th Volume, STP 1582, Robert J. Johnson, Ed., pp. 22–36, http://dx.doi.org/10.1520/STP158220140079, ASTM International, West Conshohocken, PA 2015.
19. Sulheim S, Holme I, Ekeland A, et al. Helmet use and risk of head injuries in alpine skiers and snowboarders. JAMA 2006;295:919–24.
20. Macnab AJ, Smith T, Gagnon FA, et al. Effect of helmet wear on the incidence of head/face and cervical spine injuries in young skiers and snowboarders. Inj Prev 2002;8:324–7.
21. Russell K, Christie J, Hagel BE. The effect of helmets on the risk of head and neck injuries among skiers and snowboarders: a meta-analysis. CMAJ 2010;182:333–40.
22. Rughani AI, Lin CT, Ares WJ, et al. Helmet use and reduction in skull fractures in skiers and snowboarders admitted to the hospital. J Neurosurg Pediatr 2011;7:268–71.
23. Russell K, Hagel B, Francescutti LH. The effect of wrist guards on wrist and arm injuries among snowboarders: a systematic review. Clin J Sport Med 2007;17:145–50.

24. Shuman KM, Meyers MC. Skateboarding injuries: an updated review. Phys Sportsmed 2015;43(3):317–23.
25. Safekids.org. Bicycle, Skate and Skateboard Safety Factsheet (2015) [Internet]. 2015 [cited 2015 Aug 3]; Available at: http://www.safekids.org/sites/default/files/documents/skw_bike_fact_sheet_feb_2015.pdf.
26. Kyle SB, Nance ML, Rutherford GW Jr, et al. Skateboard-associated injuries: participation-based estimates and injury characteristics. J Trauma 2002;53:686–90.
27. Keays G, Dumas A. Longboard and skateboard injuries. Injury 2014;45:1215–9.
28. Macdonald DJ, McGlone S, Exton A, et al. A new skatepark: the impact on the local hospital. Injury 2006;37:238–42.
29. Everett WW. Skatepark injuries and the influence of skatepark design: a one year consecutive case series. J Emerg Med 2002;23:269–74.
30. Rethnam U, Yesupalan RS, Sinha A. Skateboards: are they really perilous? a retrospective study from a district hospital. BMC Res Notes 2008;1:59.
31. Lustenberger T, Talving P, Barmparas G, et al. Skateboard-related injuries: not to be taken lightly. A National Trauma Databank Analysis. J Trauma 2010;69:924–7.
32. Forsman L, Eriksson A. Skateboarding injuries of today. Br J Sports Med 2001;35:325–8.
33. Shehab R, Mirabelli MH. Evaluation and diagnosis of wrist pain: a case-based approach. Am Fam Physician 2013;87:568–73.
34. Alshryda S, Shah A, Odak S, et al. Acute fractures of the scaphoid bone: systematic review and meta-analysis. Surgeon 2012;10:218–29.
35. Skateboard injuries. American Academy of Pediatrics Committee on Injury and Poison Prevention. Pediatrics 1995;95:611–2.
36. Kroncke EL, Niedfeldt MW, Young CC. Use of protective equipment by adolescents in inline skating, skateboarding, and snowboarding. Clin J Sport Med 2008;18:38–43.
37. Wu BC, Oakes JM. A randomized controlled trial of sport helmet interventions in a pediatric emergency department. Pediatr Emerg Care 2005;21:730–5.
38. Sunshine S. Surfing injuries. Curr Sports Med Rep 2003;2:136–41.
39. Nathanson A, Bird S, Dao L, et al. Competitive surfing injuries: a prospective study of surfing-related injuries among contest surfers. Am J Sports Med 2007;35:113–7.
40. Hay CS, Barton S, Sulkin T. Recreational surfing injuries in Cornwall, United Kingdom. Wilderness Environ Med 2009;20:335–8.
41. Taylor DM, Bennett D, Carter M, et al. Acute injury and chronic disability resulting from surfboard riding. J Sci Med Sport 2004;7:429–37.
42. Nathanson A, Haynes P, Galanis D. Surfing injuries. Am J Emerg Med 2002;20:155–60.
43. Taylor KS, Zoltan TB, Achar SA. Medical illnesses and injuries encountered during surfing. Curr Sports Med Rep 2006;5:262–7.
44. Zoumalan CI, Blumenkranz MS, McCulley TJ, et al. Severe surfing-related ocular injuries: the Stanford Northern Californian experience. Br J Sports Med 2008;42:855–7.
45. Kim JW, McDonald HR, Rubsamen PE, et al. Surfing-related ocular injuries. Retina 1998;18:424–9.
46. Lennon P, Murphy C, Fennessy B, et al. Auditory canal exostoses in Irish surfers. Ir J Med Sci 2015. [Epub ahead of print].

47. Attlmayr B, Smith IM. Prevalence of 'surfer's ear' in Cornish surfers. J Laryngol Otol 2015;129:440–4.
48. Kroon DF, Lawson ML, Derkay CS, et al. Surfer's ear: external auditory exostoses are more prevalent in cold water surfers. Otolaryngol Head Neck Surg 2002;126: 499–504.
49. Wong BJ, Cervantes W, Doyle KJ, et al. Prevalence of external auditory canal exostoses in surfers. Arch Otolaryngol Head Neck Surg 1999;125:969–72.
50. Sano A, Yotsumoto T. Chest injuries related to surfing. Asian Cardiovasc Thorac Ann 2015;23(7):839–41.
51. Nakamoto BK, Siu AM, Hashiba KA, et al. Surfer's myelopathy: a radiologic study of 23 cases. AJNR Am J Neuroradiol 2013;34:2393–8.
52. Aoki M, Moriizumi S, Toki M, et al. Rehabilitation and long-term course of nontraumatic myelopathy associated with surfing. Am J Phys Med Rehabil 2013;92: 828–32.
53. Chung HY, Sun SF, Wang JL, et al. Non-traumatic anterior spinal cord infarction in a novice surfer: a case report. J Neurol Sci 2011;302:118–20.
54. Lin CY, Fu JH, Li SC, et al. Surfer's myelopathy. QJM 2012;105:373–4.
55. Thompson TP, Pearce J, Chang G, et al. Surfer's myelopathy. Spine 2004;29: E353–6.
56. Aviles-Hernandez I, Garcia-Zozaya I, DeVillasante JM. Nontraumatic myelopathy associated with surfing. J Spinal Cord Med 2007;30:288–93.
57. Taylor DM, Bennett D, Carter M, DeVillasante JM. Perceptions of surfboard riders regarding need for protective headgear. Wilderness Environ Med 2005;16:75–80.
58. Jain AK, Gaynon M. Images in clinical medicine. Macular hemorrhage from bungee jumping. N Engl J Med 2007;357:e3.
59. Manos D, Hamer O, Muller NL. Pulmonary hemorrhage resulting from bungee jumping. J Thorac Imaging 2007;22:358–9.
60. Diniz JR, Arantes TE, Urbano RV, et al. Ocular alterations associated with bungee jumping: case report. Arq Bras Oftalmol 2005;68:853–6 [in Portuguese].
61. Curtis EBC, Collin HB. Ocular injury due to bungee jumping. Clin Exp Optom 1999;82:193–5.
62. Van Rens E. Traumatic ocular haemorrhage related to bungee jumping. Br J Ophthalmol 1994;78:984.
63. Jain BK, Talbot EM. Bungee jumping and intraocular haemorrhage. Br J Ophthalmol 1994;78:236–7.
64. Filipe JA, Pinto AM, Rosas V, et al. Retinal complications after bungee jumping. Int Ophthalmol 1994;18:359–60.
65. David DB, Mears T, Quinlan MP. Ocular complications associated with bungee jumping. Br J Ophthalmol 1994;78:234–5.
66. Chan J. Ophthalmic complications after bungee jumping. Br J Ophthalmol 1994; 78:239.
67. Zhou W, Huynh TT, Kougias P, et al. Traumatic carotid artery dissection caused by bungee jumping. J Vasc Surg 2007;46:1044–6.
68. FitzGerald JJ, Bassi S, White BD. A subdural haematoma following 'reverse' bungee jumping. Br J Neurosurg 2002;16:307–8.
69. Huang KW, Huang SJ, Lin TH, et al. Anterior dislocation of the humeral head from bungee jumping. Am J Emerg Med 2001;19:322–4.
70. Omololu AB, Travlos J. Bungee jumping causing a comminuted proximal femoral fracture. Injury 1995;26:413–4.
71. Torre PR, Williams GG, Blackwell T, et al. Bungee jumper's foot drop peroneal nerve palsy caused by bungee cord jumping. Ann Emerg Med 1993;22:1766–7.

72. Hite PR, Greene KA, Levy DI, et al. Injuries resulting from bungee-cord jumping. Ann Emerg Med 1993;22:1060–3.
73. Shapiro MJ, Marts B, Berni A, et al. The perils of bungee jumping. J Emerg Med 1995;13:629–31.
74. Mei-Dan O. BASE jumping. In: Mei-Dan OCM, editor. Adventure and extreme sports injuries: epidemiology, treatment, rehabilitation and prevention. London: Springer; 2013. p. 91–112.
75. Wolf BCH, Harding BE. Patterns of injury in a fatal BASE jumping accident. Am J Forensic Med Pathol 2008;29:369–451.
76. Mei-Dan O, Carmont MR, Monasterio E. The epidemiology of severe and catastrophic injuries in BASE jumping. Clin J Sport Med 2012;22:262–7.
77. Monasterio E, Mei-Dan O. Risk and severity of injury in a population of BASE jumpers. N Z Med J 2008;121:70–5.
78. Soreide K, Ellingsen CL, Knutson V. How dangerous is BASE jumping? An analysis of adverse events in 20,850 jumps from the Kjerag Massif, Norway. J Trauma 2007;62:1113–7.
79. Westman A, Rosen M, Berggren P, et al. Parachuting from fixed objects: descriptive study of 106 fatal events in BASE jumping 1981-2006. Br J Sports Med 2008; 42:431–6.
80. Schoen RG, Stano MJ. Year 2000 whitewater injury survey. Wilderness Environ Med 2002;13:119–24.
81. Fiore DC, Houston JD. Injuries in whitewater kayaking. Br J Sports Med 2001;35: 235–41.
82. Whisman SA, Hollenhorst SJ. Injuries in commercial whitewater rafting. Clin J Sport Med 1999;9:18–23.
83. Wilson I, McDermott H, Munir F, et al. Injuries, ill-health and fatalities in white water rafting and white water paddling. Sports Med 2013;43:65–75.
84. Fiore DC. Injuries associated with whitewater rafting and kayaking. Wilderness Environ Med 2003;14:255–60.
85. Centers for Disease Control and Prevention, 1997. Outbreak of leptospirosis among white-water rafters - Costa Rica, 1996. MMWR Morb Mortal Wkly Rep 46:577–9.
86. Sejvar JB, Bancroft E, Winthrop K, et al. Leptospirosis in "Eco-Challenge" athletes, Malaysian Borneo, 2000. Emerg Infect Dis 2003;9:702–7.
87. Appleton CC, Bailey IW. Canoeists and waterborne diseases in South Africa. S Afr Med J 1990;78:323–6.
88. Tebruegge M, Connell T, Ritz N, et al. *Mycobacterium marinum* infection following kayaking injury. Int J Infect Dis 2010;14(Suppl 3):e305–6.
89. Moore RD, Schuman TA, Scott TA, et al. Exostoses of the external auditory canal in white-water kayakers. Laryngoscope 2010;120:582–90.
90. Whitman L. American Whitewater - Whitewater is safer than you think. American Whitewater; 2006. Available at: https://www.americanwhitewater.org/content/Article/view/articleid/1614/. Accessed August 5, 2015.
91. Centers for Disease Control and Prevention (CDC). Paddle sports fatalities–Maine, 2000-2007. MMWR Morb Mortal Wkly Rep 2008;57:524–7.
92. Stemberga V, Cuculic D, Petaros A, et al. Kayaking fatalities: could more appropriate helmets prevent fatal consequences? Sports Med 2013;43:1201–2.

Illness in the Returned International Traveler

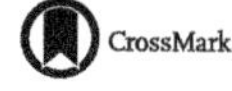

Christopher A. Sanford, MD, MPH, DTM&H[a,*], Claire Fung, MD, MPH[b,c]

KEYWORDS

- Post-travel illness • Travel medicine • Gastrointestinal • Diarrhea • Fever
- Dermatology • Infectious disease • Eosinophilia

KEY POINTS

- Illness is common in travelers to low-income nations: between 20% and 70% of travelers to low-income nations become ill during or after their trip.
- The most common 3 categories of illness in international travelers are gastrointestinal, fever, and dermatoses.
- Familiarity with the epidemiology, mode of transmission, and risk factors for acquisition for common infectious illnesses can facilitate work-up of illness in returned international travelers.

INTRODUCTION

International travel increases each year. International tourist arrivals increased from 25 million in 1950 to 1 billion in 2012, and are anticipated to increase to 1.8 billion by 2030.[1,2] Illness in international travelers is common. Between 20% and 70% of travelers from high-income nations to low-income nations report travel-associated illness; 1% to 5% become sufficiently ill as to seek medical attention during or after travel; between 1 in 1000 and 1 in 10,000 require medical evacuation, and 1 in 100,000 dies.[3,4]

Medical providers are increasingly likely to see patients who have acquired illnesses abroad and should be aware of illnesses associated with specific itineraries, activities, and exposures. The 3 most common categories of illnesses in returned international travelers are gastrointestinal, fever, and dermatologic disorders. In a study of 42,173 ill returned international travelers seen at post-travel clinics between 2007 and 2011, 34.0% were seen for gastrointestinal disease, 23.3% were seen for fever, and 19.5% were seen for dermatologic disorder; these 3 categories accounted for three-quarters of travel-related diseases.[5]

[a] Family Medicine, Global Health, University of Washington, Box 358732, Seattle, WA 98125, USA; [b] Family Medicine, The Everett Clinic at Snohomish, 401 2nd Street, Snohomish, WA 98290, USA; [c] Department of Family Medicine, University of Washington Family Medicine Residency, 331 Northeast Thornton Place, Seattle, WA 98125, USA
* Corresponding author.
E-mail address: casanfo@uw.edu

Med Clin N Am 100 (2016) 393–409
http://dx.doi.org/10.1016/j.mcna.2015.08.016 medical.theclinics.com

GASTROINTESTINAL DISORDERS IN THE RETURNING TRAVELER

Pathophysiology

Diarrhea is the most common illness reported in returned international travelers.[5] Traveler's diarrhea (TD) is defined as 3 or more unformed stools per day plus other gastrointestinal symptoms, such as abdominal pain, associated with travel. Risk factors include young age, adventurous travel (trekking, camping, and safaris), travel to tropical climates, higher socioeconomic status, and medical conditions resulting in immunocompromised state or decreased gastric acidity.[6] Attack rates of TD range from 30% to 70% of travelers, depending on destination.[7]

TD can be separated into 2 categories: classical TD and persistent/protracted TD (PTD). Because it is brief in duration and a majority of cases resolve within the first week of travel, classical TD is not usually evaluated in a physician's office. PTD is travel-acquired diarrhea that is longer in duration (>14 days) after returning from travel and may require evaluation by a physician.[8]

Clinical Presentation

Classical TD is typically mild, with an average of 4.6 stools per day and complaints of nausea and abdominal pain. Classical TD is also self-limited and typically diarrhea resolves within 3 to 5 days without antibiotic treatment. PTD can often include fever and bloody diarrhea. Severe disease may lead to orthostatic hemodynamic instability from inability to maintain oral hydration.

Patient History

A detailed history of present illness, including onset, associated symptoms, and duration, is important in determining the cause of TD. Symptom severity and presence or absence of blood or mucus in the stool may be suggestive of certain pathogens over others, although it is important to note any history of or possible exacerbations of other chronic gastrointestinal disorders, such as irritable bowel syndrome or inflammatory bowel disease.

Physical Examination

In classical TD, abdominal examination typically reveals a soft, nontender, or minimally diffusely tender abdomen with hyperactive bowel sounds. In PTD, rectal examination may be useful to rule out diarrhea around impacted stool from use of antimotility agents and dehydration, or to exclude other noninfectious causes of gross blood in the stool, such as rectal hemorrhoids or anal fissure.

Diagnostic Testing

Laboratory studies may be indicated in returning international travelers presenting with diarrhea depending on the duration and severity of illness. Classical TD is most commonly caused by enterotoxigenic strains of *Escherichia coli*. Enterotoxigenic *E coli*, *Salmonella*, *Shigella*, and *Campylobacter* account for 45% to 50% of cases of TD. Viruses and protozoa account for 5% to 10% of cases, and in 30% of cases of TD, no pathogen is identified.[9] **Table 1** lists diagnostic stool tests that may be useful in identifying the cause of diarrhea in the returned traveler. Stool tests are helpful when positive; however, they tend to lack sensitivity.

Some limited blood testing may be helpful in patients presenting with PTD. A complete blood cell count with differential may be indicative of bacterial infection if it shows leukocytosis with neutrophilia. Marked leukocytosis (>20,000 cells/dL) should raise concern for *Clostridium difficile* infection. Eosinophilia can be suggestive of parasitic or invasive helminthic infection. Other blood tests can be used to explore other

Table 1
Diagnostic stool tests for returned travelers with diarrhea

Diagnostic Procedure	Indication
Direct examination of stool	Blood in stool suggests inflammatory process Greasy/frothy stool suggests malabsorption
Stool white blood cells	Presence of multiple stool white blood cells suggests bacterial infection
Stool ova and parasites	Detect helminth eggs and larvae Detect protozoan cysts and trophozoites
Stool Gram stain	Comma-shaped organisms suggest *Campylobacter*
Stool wet preparation	Detects live actively mobile protozoan trophozoites
Stool bacterial culture	Detects bacterial enteric pathogens, including *Salmonella, Shigella, Campylobacter*
Stool acid-fast stain	Detects *Cryptosporidium*
Stool trichrome blue stain	Detects microsporidia
Stool safranin stain	Detects *Cyclospora*
Enzyme-linked immunoassay	Separate assays specifically used for detection of *Giardia, Cryptosporidium, E coli* O157:H7, *Entamoeba histolytica, C difficile*

Adapted from Rosenblatt JE. Approach to Diarrhea in Returned Travelers. Jong EC, Sanford C. The travel and tropical medicine manual. 4th edition. New York: Elsevier; 2008; with permission.

causes of diarrhea, such as hyperthyroidism, systemic inflammation, and nutritional deficiencies causing malabsorption.[10]

Management Goals

Primary management of TD should focus on rehydration. Treatment should be based on the cause of the disease.

Self-management Strategies

Classical TD is self-limited and usually self-managed by the traveler while abroad. Empiric self-treatment with antimicrobials typically shortens the course of classical TD to 1 day, compared with 3 to 5 days if left untreated. Self-treatment with antimicrobials also tends to reduce associated symptoms such as abdominal cramping.[11]

Travelers returning from Africa or Latin America are typically treated with a fluoroquinolone, such as ciprofloxacin. Travelers returning from Southeast or South Asia should be treated with a macrolide, such as azithromycin, due to increasing resistance of *Campylobacter* and *Shigella* species to fluoroquinolones. Self-treatment of TD among adults may also include antimotility agents (such as loperamide) as well as oral rehydration solution, in addition to empiric antibiotics Antimotility agents remain contraindicated in children under 3 years of age and should also be avoided if there is evidence of dysentery (fever or bloody diarrhea).[12] As a general rule, the faster the diet is advanced from fluids only, the faster the recovery. Data remain mixed on effectiveness of diet restriction (avoidance of dairy, fruit juices, concentrated sweets, and high-fat foods) in symptomatic treatment of TD.[13]

Pharmacologic Strategies

Tables 2–4 list treatments of specific causes of TD. Empiric treatment with antimicrobials can be used as both a diagnostic and therapeutic tool in treatment of PTD. A

Table 2
Common bacterial causes of diarrhea in returned travelers

Bacterial Etiologic Agent	Incubation Period	Signs and Symptoms	Duration of Illness	Possible Exposures	Laboratory Testing	Treatment/Management
Campylobacter jejuni	2–5 d	Diarrhea (±blood), cramps, fever, vomiting	2–10 d	Uncooked poultry, unpasteurized milk, contaminated water	Stool culture	Supportive care. • Erythromycin and quinolones may be indicated early in diarrheal disease
Clostridium difficile	3–7 d	Diarrhea, fever, cramps	Days – several weeks	Antibiotics	*C difficile* toxin stool culture	Metronidazole or po vancomycin
Enterohemorrhagic *E coli*, including *E coli O157:H7*	1–8 d	Severe (often bloody) diarrhea, abdominal pain, vomiting	5–10 d	Uncooked beef, unpasteurized milk/juice, raw fruits and vegetables, contaminated water	Stool culture (if *E coli* 0157:H7 is suspected, specific testing must be requested)	Supportive care • Monitor renal function, hemoglobin, and platelets • Associated with HUS
Enterotoxigenic *E coli*	1–3 d	Watery diarrhea, cramps, some vomiting	3–7 d	Fecal-oral	Stool culture (if suspected, must request specific testing)	Supportive care Antibiotics (TMP-SMX or quinolones) in severe cases
Salmonella spp	1–3 d	Diarrhea, fever, cramps, vomiting	4–7 d	Contaminated eggs, poultry, unpasteurized milk/juice/cheese, contaminated raw fruits and vegetables	Stool culture	Supportive care • Antibiotics (TMP-SMX, ampicillin, gentamycin or quinolones) only indicated for extraintestinal spread
Shigella spp	1–2 d	Diarrhea (±blood or mucus), cramps, fever	4–7 d	Fecal-oral	Stool cultures	Quinolones

Vibrio cholerae (toxin)	1–3 d	Profuse watery diarrhea and vomiting; severe dehydration	3–7 d	Contaminated water, fish, shellfish, street-vended food typically from Latin America or Asia	Stool culture (if suspected, must request specific testing)	Supportive care with aggressive oral and intravenous rehydration • If confirmed, tetracycline or doxycycline for adults, TMP-SMX for children <8 yo
Vibrio parahaemolyticus	2 h–2 d	Water diarrhea, cramps, nausea/vomiting	2–5 d	Uncooked fish/shellfish	Stool cultures (if suspected, must request specific testing)	Supportive care • Antibiotics (tetracycline, doxycycline, gentamicin, and cefotaxime) if severe
Vibrio vulnificus	1–7 d	Diarrhea, vomiting, abdominal pain, bacteremia, and wound infections. More common in immunocompromised or patients with chronic liver disease	2–8 d	Uncooked shellfish, especially oysters and open wounds exposed to sea water	Stool, wound, or blood cultures (if suspected, must request specific testing)	Supportive care and antibiotics (tetracycline or doxycycline, plus ceftazidime)
Yersinia enterocolytica	1–2 d	Diarrhea, vomiting, fever, abdominal pain. More common in older children and young adults	1–3 wk	Uncooked pork, unpasteurized milk/tofu, contaminated water	Stool/vomitus/blood culture (if suspected, must request specific testing) Serology available in research reference laboratories	Supportive care • Antibiotics (gentamicin or cefotaxime) if septicemia occurs

Abbreviations: HUS, hemolytic uremic syndrome; TMP-SMX, trimethoprim/sulfamethoxazole; yo, years old.

From American Medical Association; American Nurses Association-American Nurses Foundation; Centers for Disease Control and Prevention; et al. Diagnosis and management of foodborne illnesses: a primer for physicians and other health care professionals. MMWR Recomm Rep 2004;53(RR-4):1–33.

Table 3
Common viral causes of diarrhea in returned travelers

Viral Etiologic Agent	Incubation Period	Signs and Symptoms	Duration of Illness	Possible Exposures	Laboratory Testing	Treatment
Norovirus	0.5–2 d	Diarrhea (more common in adults), nausea, vomiting, cramps, fever, myalgias	0.5–2.5 d	Shellfish, fecal-oral	Polymerase chain reaction and electron microscopy on fresh unpreserved stool, clinical diagnosis, absence of white blood cells in stool	Supportive care

Table 4
Common parasitic causes of diarrhea in returned travelers

Parasitic Etiologic Agent	Incubation Period	Signs and Symptoms	Duration of Illness	Possible Exposures	Laboratory Testing	Treatment
Cryptosporidium	2–10 d	Diarrhea (usually watery), cramps, low-grade fever	May be relapsing and remitting over weeks to months	Uncooked food or contaminated food by an ill food handler	Specific examination of stool for *Cryptosporidium*	Supportive care, self-limited • If severe, consider paromomycin × 7 d for adults or nitazoxanide × 3 d for children 1–11 yo
Cyclospora cayetanensis	1–14 d	Diarrhea (usually watery), loss of appetite, substantial weight loss, cramps, nausea, vomiting, fatigue	May be relapsing and remitting over weeks to months	Various types of fresh produce	Specific examination of stool for *Cyclospora*	TMP-SMX × 7 d
Entamoeba histolytica	2 d – 4 wk	Diarrhea (often bloody), lower abdomen pain	May last several weeks to several months	Uncooked food or food contaminated by an ill food handler	Stool examination for cysts and parasites (may need at least 3 samples), serology for long-term infections	Metronidazole + iodoquinol or paromomycin
Giardia lamblia	1–2 wk	Diarrhea, cramps, gas, bloating	Days to weeks	Uncooked food or food contaminated by an ill food handler	Stool examination for ova and parasites (may need at least 3 samples)	Metronidazole
Trichinella spiralis	1–2 d for initial symptoms, others begin 2–8 wk after infection	Diarrhea, nausea, vomiting, fatigue, fever, abdominal discomfort, followed by myalgias, weakness and occasional cardiac and neurologic complications	Months	Uncooked contaminated meat (usually pork or wild game)	Serology	Mebendazole or albendazole

flouroquinolone or a macrolide can be used, as discussed previously. Similarly, a treatment dose of tinidazole (2 g once by mouth) may be used if giardiasis is suspected.

FEVER

Fever is reported by 2% to 3% of US and European travelers who visit low-income nations.[14,15] According to data from GeoSentinel, a network of 59 travel clinics around the world, the most common cause of fever is malaria (29%), followed by dengue fever (15%). Malaria is disproportionately diagnosed in those returned from Africa, whereas dengue fever is more common in those returning from Southeast Asia, Latin America, and the Caribbean. Other common causes of fever include enteric fever (typhoid and paratyphoid), chikungunya fever, rickettsial diseases, viral hepatitis (primarily A and B), leptospirosis, tuberculosis, and acute HIV. Typhoid fever, also known as enteric fever, is more common in those returning from South Asia; spotted fever rickettsiosis has been found in 6% of those with fever returning from sub-Saharan Africa (most commonly South Africa). In almost 40% of returned travelers with fever, no cause of the fever is identified. Causes of fever from 3 published series are listed in **Table 5**.

Fever in the returned international traveler is a marker of significant and potentially life-threatening illness. A study of more than 80,000 ill returned travelers found that 4.4% had fever. Significantly, 91% of those with potentially life-threatening illnesses had fever. The most common diagnoses were falciparum malaria (76.9%), typhoid fever (18.1%), and leptospirosis (2.4%). Among the 13 patients who died, 10 had falciparum malaria, 2 had meloidosis, and 1 had severe dengue fever. Risk factors for falciparum malaria were being male, visiting friends and relatives, and visiting West Africa. In this large series, no cases of yellow fever, Lassa fever, or Ebola virus disease were detected.[16]

Because fever may be a marker of an acute and potentially life-threatening illness, medical work-up of the febrile returned international traveler must be conducted

Table 5
Causes of fever from published series (United Kingdom, Canada, and Australia)

	Doherty et al,[22] 1995 (1995) % of Total	Maclean et al,[23] 1994 (587) %	O'Brien et al,[24] 2001 (232) %
Malaria	42	32	27
Respiratory tract infection (upper respiratory tract infection, pneumonia, bronchitis)	2.6	11	24
Diarrhea/dysentery	6.6	4.5	14
Dengue	6.2	2	8
Hepatitis	3 (hepatitis A only)	6	3 (hepatitis A only)
Enteric fever	1.5	2	3
Urinary tract infection/ pyelonephritis	2.6	4	2
Rickettsial	1.6	1	2
Tuberculosis	1.6	1	0.4
Amebiasis/liver abscess	0	1	1
No diagnosis	24.6	25	9

From Wilson ME, Schwartz E. Fever. In: Keystone JS, Kozarsky PE, Freedman DO, et al. editors. Travel medicine. Edinburgh (United Kingdom): Mosby; 2004; with permission.

promptly. The initial diagnostic work-up should focus on diseases that are life-threatening, treatable, or transmissible. Medical providers should have a low threshold for hospitalizing febrile returned travelers.

Obtaining a detailed history from returned febrile traveler is mandatory. Important topics to address include pretravel immunizations, itinerary, dates of travel, duration since return, activities during travel, exposure to new sexual partners, exposures to needles and blood, exposure to bodies of fresh water, animal and arthropod bites, compliance with malaria prophylaxis, and treatments, if any, to date. Specific exposures associated with febrile illnesses are provided in **Table 6**.

The timing of the onset of fever relative to travel can be useful in generating a differential diagnosis. There is a characteristic duration between exposure and fever for many causes of fever. For example, dengue fever has a brief incubation period (usually 4–7 days; range 3–14 days); hence, fever appearing in a traveler who returned from the tropics over 14 days prior is unlikely to be due to dengue. The incubation periods of several infectious diseases are listed in **Table 7**.

Table 6
Febrile conditions associated with specific exposures

Exposure	Condition
Food and water	
Unsanitary water or food	Hepatitis A or E Enteric fever (typhoid or paratyphoid) Bacterial gastroenteritis Amebiasis
Undercooked meat or fish	Hepatitis A Toxoplasmosis Trichinella
Unpasteurized milk products	Brucella Enteric fever *Salmonella* gastroenteritis Tuberculosis (bovis)
Arthropods	
Mosquitoes	Malaria Dengue fever Filariasis Loa loa Yellow fever Other arboviruses
Ticks	Tick typhus (Mediterranean or African) Rocky Mountain spotted fever Crimean-Congo hemorrhagic fever Lyme disease Relapsing fever Tularemia Babesiosis Ehrlichia
Sandflies	Leishmaniasis Sandfly fever Bartonellosis (Oroya fever)

(*continued on next page*)

Table 6
(*continued*)

Exposure	Condition
Black flies	Onchocerciasis
Tsetse flies	African trypanosomiasis
Reduvid bugs	American trypanosomiasis (Chagas disease)
Chiggers	Scrub typhus
Caves	Rabies Histoplasmosis
Western hemisphere desert area (in particular construction or archeological sites)	Coccidiomycosis
Animal exposures	Brucellosis Rabies Tularemia Q fever Anthrax Plague Viral hemorrhagic fevers
Sexual contact	HIV Hepatitis B STIs, including herpes simplex virus gonorrhea, syphilis, others
Crowded living conditions, group travel, exposure to ill persons	Meningococcal disease Influenza Tuberculosis Hepatitis A Lassa, Marburg, Ebola viruses
Fresh water (swimming or wading)	Schistosomiasis Leptospirosis Hepatitis A

Adapted from McLellan SLF. Evaluation of fever in the returned traveler. Prim Care 2002;29(4):950–1; with permission.

Table 7
Incubation periods

Short (<10 d)	Intermediate (10–21 d)	Long (>21 d)
Malaria	Malaria	Malaria
Influenza	Typhoid fever	Hepatitis A, B, C, and E
Dengue fever	Leptospirosis	Schistosomiasis (Katayama fever)
Yellow fever	Brucellosis	Leishmaniasis
Enteric bacterial infection	African trypanosomiasis	Amebic liver abscess
African tick-bite fever	Viral hemorrhagic fevers	Tuberculosis
Plague	Q fever	Filariasis
Spotted fever group, including Rocky Mountain	Relapsing fever	HIV
Spotted fever		

Adapted from Leggatt PA. Assessment of febrile illness in the returned traveler. Aust Fam Physician 2007;36(5):332.

Work-up

The laboratory work-up of the febrile returned traveler should include a complete blood cell count with differential, hepatic transaminases, renal function tests (creatinine and blood urea nitrogen), urinalysis, and chest radiograph, and, in those with a history of exposure to malaria, thick and thin smears in addition to a malaria rapid diagnostic test (eg, BinaxNOW Malaria antigen assay (Alere, Seattle, WA, USA)). In long-duration travelers, consideration should be given to testing for tuberculosis either by purified protein derivative or interferon-gamma release assay (eg, QuantiFERON-TB Gold (Qiagen, Venlo, Netherlands)). Even those with a history of compliance with an efficacious malaria prophylaxis regimen should be tested for malaria. It may be prudent to save a tube of serum to be used as an acute-phase serum for tests that clinicians may later consider. Additional tests to consider include specific serologies (dengue fever, rickettsial diseases, fungal disease, brucella, Lyme disease, arboviruses, leptospirosis, filariasis, and schistosomiasis), blood cultures, and stool studies, including ova and parasite × 3, culture and sensitivity, *Giardia* antigen, and fecal leukocytes.

An elevated eosinophil count may guide diagnosis. In high-income nations, the most common causes of eosinophilia are allergic and atopic diseases; in returned international travelers, this suggests infection with a tissue-invasive helminth. Among the helminth infections that elevate the eosinophil count are *Ascaris* (roundworm), *Strongyloides*, *Trichinella*, and *Enterobius vermicularis* (known as pinworm in the United States and threadworm in the United Kingdom.) Other parasitic infections causing eosinophilia include cysticercosis (caused by *Taenia solium*), echinococcosis, filariasis, hookworm infection, paragonimiasis, schistosomiasis, and visceral larva migrans.[17] Malaria does not cause eosinophilia. **Table 8** lists parasitic diseases in travelers, ordered by degree of eosinophilia.

Minor elevation of hepatic transaminases (2–3× upper range of normal) is nonspecific; marked elevation suggests acute viral hepatitis. The presence of fecal leukocytes suggests infection with an invasive gastrointestinal organism, for example, *Salmonella* or *Shigella*.

If a returned traveler has significant abdominal pain, clinicians should consider imaging the abdomen (ultrasound or CT) to evaluate for, among other causes of fever, amebic liver abscess.

In a stable patient, treatment of malaria should be initiated only after the diagnosis of malaria is confirmed by laboratory testing. In an unstable patient, presumptive treatment of malaria may be initiated if the clinical scenario is consistent with malaria after consultation with an infectious disease specialist.

DERMATOSES

Common causes of dermatologic symptoms in international travelers returned from the tropics include cutaneous larva migrans (CLM), pyodermas, arthropod-related pruritic dermatitis, myiasis, tungiasis, cutaneous leishmaniasis, scabies, and cutaneous fungal infections. A study of 784 US travelers to low-income nations found that 8% (63) developed skin disorders: 14 were related to insect bites or stings, 10 to sun exposure, 7 to dermatophytes, 7 to contact allergy, and 5 to infectious cellulitis.[15] In study of 269 post-travel patients who presented to a tropical disease clinic in Paris with travel-related dermatoses, a firm diagnosis was made in 97% of patients; of these, 53% involved an imported tropical disease (**Table 9**).[18]

Cutaneous Larva Migrans

CLM (also known as creeping eruption, clam digger's itch, and sand worm eruption) is the most frequent travel-associated skin disease of travelers to the tropics. Most often

Table 8
Parasitic infectious diseases in travelers, ordered by degree of eosinophilia

Disease	Eosinophilia[a]	Associated Findings
Malaria	Absent	Fever, headache, myalgia
Toxoplasmosis	Absent	Fever (in some cases), lymphadenopathy
Amebiasis	Absent	Colitis or liver abscess
Giardiasis	Absent	Diarrhea
Leishmaniasis	Absent	Cutaneous, mucocutaneous, and visceral disease; fever only in visceral disease
Ascaris lumbricoides infection (adult stage)	Absent	Intestinal infection with adult worms not associated with eosinophilia
Tapeworm infection	Absent	Intestinal infection with adult worms not associated with eosinophilia
Dientamoeba fragilis infection[b]	Absent or mild	Persistent diarrhea and (in some cases) associated enterobiasis
Trichuriasis (whipworm infection)	Absent or mild	Proctitis
Enterobiasis (pinworm infection)	Absent or mild	Perianal itching (often nocturnal)
Schistosomiasis	Absent or mild; may be moderate to high in acute schistosomiasis (Katayama fever)	Intestinal, hepatic, and bladder abnormalities; fever in acute schistosomiasis (Katayama fever)
Cysticercosis (*Taenia solium* infection, larval stage)	Absent or mild; may be moderate if encysted larvae die and release antigen	Subcutaneous and central nervous system cysts
Echinococcosis (hydatid disease)	Absent or mild; may increase in severity if cysts rupture or leak	Cysts (hepatic, lung, bone, or other)
Chronic clonorchiasis and opisthorchiasis	Absent or mild; may be moderate or marked in early infection	Recurrent cholangitis
Isosporiasis[b]	Absent (in immunocompromised persons) or mild	Chronic diarrhea in immunocompromised persons
Paragonimiasis	Absent or mild; moderate or marked during larval migration	Infection with lung fluke; pulmonary nodule; mimics TB or cancer; may cavitate
Hookworm infection	Absent or mild; moderate or marked during larval migration	Iron-deficiency anemia

Sparganosis	Absent or mild	Infection with spirometra tapeworm; swelling, edema, inflammation, mass lesion, necrosis with migrating larva
Strongyloidiasis	Absent (in disseminated infection), mild, or moderate	Intestinal infection may persist for decades
A lumbricoides infection (larval stage)	Mild or moderate	In acute infection, pulmonary migration of larvae (before oviposition)
Angiostrongyliasis (*Angiostrongylus cantonensis* infection)	Mild or moderate	Eosinophilic meningitis; fever in some cases
Gnathostomiasis	Mild, moderate, or marked	Swelling edema, inflammation, necrosis associated with migrating larva, migratory soft tissue mass, radiculomyelitis, or eosinophilic meningitis
Onchocerciasis	Mild, moderate, or marked	Subcutaneous nodules, dermatitis, and keratitis
Fascioliasis (*Fasciola hepatica* [liver fluke] infection)	Mild, moderate, or marked (during larval migration)	Acute destructive hepatic parenchymal lesions during the acute stage of larval migration; chronic biliary obstruction
Lymphatic filariasis	Mild, moderate, or marked	Retrograde lymphangitis, lymphadenopathy, soft tissue swelling or edema and rash; fever
Loiasis	Moderate or marked	Soft tissue edema (Calabar swellings) and eyeworm (associated with migration of worms)
Toxocariasis	Moderate or marked	Visceral larva migrans
Acute trichinosis	Moderate or marked	Myalgia, diffuse edema; fever in some cases
Tropical pulmonary eosinophilia (occult lymphatic filariasis)	Marked	Reactive airways, paroxysmal nocturnal dyspnea, and pulmonary infiltrates

The most characteristic levels of eosinophila associated with each infection are listed; the degree of eosinophilia in an individual patient may differ. Parasites other than those listed may cause eosinophilia. Nonparasitic infectious causes of eosinophilia include HIV, human T-cell leukemia virus type I, *Mycobacterium tuberculosis*, *Treponema pallidum*, and *Bartonella henselae*. Eosinophilia may also occur in lepromatous leprosy, resolving scarlet fever, coccidioidomycosis, and allergic bronchopulmonary aspergillosis.

[a] Eosinophila is considered absent if there are fewer than 400 eosinophils per μL of peripheral blood, mild if there are 400 to 1000 eosinophils per μL, moderate if there are 1000 to 3000 eosinophils per μL, and marked if there are more than 3000 eosinophils per μL.

[b] *D fragilis* infection and isosporiasis (due to *Isospora belli*) are the only protozoal infections that are associated with eosinophilia.

From Ryan ET, Wilson ME, Kain KC. Illness after international travel. N Engl J Med 2002;347(7):512; with permission.

Table 9
Travel-associated dermatoses diagnosed in 269 French travelers presenting to a tropical medicine clinic in Paris, 1991–1993

Diagnosis	Number of Cases (%)
Cutaneous larva migrans	65 (24.9)
Pyodermas	48 (17.8)
Arthropod-related pruritic dermatitis	26 (9.7)
Myiasis	25 (9.3)
Tungiasis	17 (6.3)
Urticaria	16 (5.9)
Rash with fever	11 (4.1)
Cutaneous leishmaniasis	8 (3.0)
Scabies	6 (2.2)
Injuries[a]	5 (1.9)
Cutaneous fungal infections	5 (1.9)
Exacerbation of preexisting illness	5 (1.9)
Sexually transmitted disease	4 (1.5)
Cutaneous herpes simplex	3 (1.1)
Septicemia	3 (1.1)
Acute venous thrombosis	2 (0.7)
Pityriasis rosea	2 (0.7)
Mycobacterium marinum infection	2 (0.7)
Acute lymphatic filariasis	1 (0.4)
Traumatic abrasion	1 (0.4)
Miscellaneous[b]	3 (1.1)
Undetermined	9 (3.3)
Total	269 (100)

[a] Injuries included local envenomation (1 case), superficial injuries caused by contact with marine creatures (2 cases), and cellulitis-like reactions presumably caused by arthropods (2 cases).
[b] Miscellaneous diagnoses were lichen planus, erythema nodosum (manifesting infection with *Salmonella enteritidis*, and Reiter syndrome (of unknown cause).

caused by the larvae of hookworms (*Ancyclostoma* species) of dogs, cats, and other mammals, this condition has a worldwide distribution in the tropics and subtropics. It is transmitted by skin contact with infective larvae in beach sand or soil, usually while walking barefoot, sitting, or lying on beaches or soil.

The incubation period is usually 1 to 5 days but rarely can be more than a month.

CLM typically presents as a serpiginous, erythematous track associated with intense itching and mild swelling. Typical locations are the feet, buttocks, and, more rarely, trunk or other locations.[19] The track advances from a few millimeters to a few centimeters each day as the larvae migrate.

This infestation usually spontaneously resolves, usually within weeks to months. The treatment of choice is albendazole (400 mg orally daily for 3 days). Cryotherapy is often ineffective because the larva may be up to 2 cm ahead of the visible burrow.

Risk of acquiring CLM is reduced by wearing protective footwear while walking on beaches or soil and by not sitting or lying on beaches or soil.

Localized Cutaneous Leishmaniasis

Leishmaniasis is infection with protozoan *Leishmania* species, for which the vector is the phlebotamine sandfly. Travelers may not notice sandfly bites, because sandflies are silent and small (approximately one-third the size of mosquitoes or smaller); bites may be painless. In addition to cutaneous leishmaniasis, the *Leishmania* parasite can cause visceral leishmaniasis, which affects spleen, liver, and bone marrow.

Localized cutaneous leishmaniasis (LCL) is transmitted in almost 100 tropical and warm temperate countries. New World LCL is transmitted in forested regions of Latin America; it is usually caused by species of *L braziliensis* and *L mexicana* complexes. Old World LCL, most commonly caused by *L major* and *L tropica*, occurs in sub-Saharan and North Africa, the Mediterranean basin, and regions of the Middle East.

US tourists most commonly acquire this infection in Central and South America.

Initial prevalence rates in US military personnel deployed to the Middle East were high, with more than 600 cases of leishmaniasis in personnel deployed to Iraq in 2003. The marked decline in cases seen subsequently was probably due to improvements in housing for military personnel, control of sandflies, and increased use of personal protection measures.[20]

Clinical forms of LCL include papule, nodule, plaque, ulcer, and nodular lymphangitis; of these forms, cutaneous ulcer is the most frequent clinical presentation of New World LCL. Ulcers usually have a well-circumscribed border and a crusted base; they are painless. Mucocutaneous leishmaniasis most commonly occurs in South America. It is a more destructive form of leishmaniasis, causing erosion of the palate, nasal septum, lips, and adjacent tissues. It is rare in travelers.

Diagnosis is most commonly made with skin biopsy from the ulcer edge. The resulting slit-skin smears are grown on various media, stained with Giemsa, and examined under light microscopy for the characteristic amastigotes (tissue stage of the parasite.)

The mainstay of treatment is liposomal amphotericin, which has largely replaced the pentavalent antimonial agents sodium stibogluconate (Pentostam) and meglumine antimonate (Glucantime) as first-line therapy. Management of these conditions may be challenging, and they should usually be treated by an expert.

Myiasis

Cutaneous myiasis is skin infestation with fly larva; it is most frequently caused by the tumbu fly (*Cordylobia anthropophaga*) in sub-Saharan Africa and by the bot fly (*Dermatobia hominis*) in Central and South America. Tumbu fly larvae penetrate the skin after hatching from eggs on clothing and linens, usually after drying on clothing lines. Lesions typically appear on body locations covered by clothing. Bot fly larvae are deposited on the skin by mosquitoes; lesions are more common on uncovered areas of skin. The incubation period for larva from the tumbu fly is 7 to 10 days; for the bot fly it is 15 to 45 days.

The skin lesions of both these myiases consists of a 1-cm to 2-cm furuncular swelling with a minor central punctum that discharges a small amount of serosanguineous or purulent fluid. The patient usually complains of a sense of movement within the lesion; often this is painful. The number of lesions is typically higher for those with tumbu fly myiasis than with bot fly myiasis: in 1 study of travelers with myiasis, the patients with tumbu fly myiasis had, on average, 5 lesions, whereas those with bot fly myiasis had 1.7 lesions.[21]

Treatment of myiasis is removal of the larvae. Tumbu fly larvae can be expressed from skin by firm lateral pressure to either side of the lesion. Bot fly larvae extraction involves first placing an occlusive substance (eg, petroleum jelly or bacon fat) over the lesion. Over ensuing hours, the larvae migrate toward the surface of the skin, facilitating removal. A snake venom extractor (syringe with adaptor to create a vacuum over the skin) has been used by some providers for more rapid results. Although most travelers are fundamentally creeped out by having wriggling larvae in their skin, significant morbidity, aside from local cellulitis, is rare.

Tumbu fly myiasis can be prevented by ironing clothing and linens after they are dried on a clothing line. Risk of bot fly myiasis can be reduced by covering skin while outdoors, the application of *N, N-Diethyl-meta*-toluamide (DEET) or picaridin to exposed skin, applying permethrin to clothing, and sleeping under a permethrin-treated bed net.

Other common causes of dermatologic disorders in international travelers include tungiasis (sand flea infestation, most commonly presenting on the feet, often adjacent to a toenail), pyodermas (bacterial skin infections, often secondary to insect bites), dermatophytoses (tinea corporis or ringworm, which is more common in the tropics and subtropics), and arthropod-related dermatoses.

OTHER CAUSES OF ILLNESS IN RETURNED INTERNATIONAL TRAVELERS

After gastrointestinal disorders, fever, and dermatoses, the 3 most common categories of illnesses in returned international travelers are respiratory or pharyngeal disorders (11%); genitourinary, sexually transmitted infections, and gynecologic disorders (3%); and neurologic disorders (2%.) The most common respiratory and pharyngeal illnesses are nonspecific upper respiratory infections, influenza, influenza-like illnesses, bronchitis, and pneumonia. The most common neurologic disorder in returned international travelers is ciguatera intoxication, which results from the consumption of contaminated reef fish; it is associated with a syndrome of paresthesia, nerve palsy, and hot/cold temperature reversal that may persist for weeks. Other neurologic disorders seen in returned travelers include neurocysticercosis, TB meningitis or tuberculoma, scombroid, and neurotoxic or paralytic shellfish poisoning.[5]

An important caveat for medical providers who care for returned international travelers to bear in mind is that a significant proportion of illness in the post-travel period is unrelated to travel. Hence, when clinicians generate differential diagnoses for given symptoms, they should include both travel-related and domestic causes.

REFERENCES

1. United Nations World Tourism Organization (UNWTO) web site Available at: http://www2.unwto.org/?q=facts/wtb.html. Accessed April 28, 2013.
2. United Nations World Tourism Organization (UNWTO) online document Tourism Market Trends. Available at: http://dtxtq4w60xqpw.cloudfront.net/sites/all/files/docpdf/markettrends.pdf. Accessed April 28, 2013.
3. Steffen R, Rickenbach M, Wilhelm U, et al. Health problems after travel to developing countries. J Infect Dis 1987;156:84–91.
4. Ryan ET, Kain KC. Health advice and immunizations for travelers. N Engl J Med 2000;342:1716–25.
5. Leder K, Torresi J, Libman MD, et al. GeoSentinel surveillance of illness in returned travelers, 2007–2011. Ann Intern Med 2013;158(6):456–68.
6. Steffen R. Epidemiology of traveler's diarrhea. Clin Infect Dis 2005;41(Suppl 8): S536–40.
7. Centers for Disease Control and Prevention. CDC health information for international travel 2012. Traveler's Diarrhea. New York: Oxford University Press; 2016.

8. International Working Group on Persistent Diarrhea. Evaluation of an algorithm for the treatment of persistent diarrhea: a multicenter study. Bull World Health Organ 1996;74:478.
9. Black RE. Epidemiology of travelers' diarrhea and relative importance of various pathogens. Rev Infect Dis 1990;12:S73–9.
10. de Saussure PP. Management of the returning traveler with diarrhea. Therap Adv Gastroenterol 2009;2(6):367–75.
11. De Bruyn G, Hahn S, Borwick A, et al. Review antibiotic treatment for travellers' diarrhoea. Cochrane Database Syst Rev 2000;(3):CD002242.
12. Li ST, Grossman DC, Cummings P. Loperamide therapy for acute diarrhea in children: systematic review and meta-analysis. PLoS Med 2007;4(3):e98.
13. Huang DB, Awasthi M, Le BM, et al. The role of diet in the treatment of travelers' diarrhea: a pilot study. Clin Infect Dis 2004;39(4):468–71.
14. Wilson MD, Pearson R. Fever and systemic symptoms. In: Guerrant FL, Walker DH, Weller PF, editors. Tropical infectious diseases. Principles, pathogens, and practice. Philadelphia: Churchill Livingston; 1999. p. 1381–99.
15. Hill DR. Health problems in a large cohort of American traveling to developing countries. J Travel Med 2000;7:259–66.
16. Jensenius M, Han PV, Schlagenhauf P, et al. Acute and potentially life-threatening tropical diseases in western travelers: a GeoSentinel multicenter study, 1996-2011. Am J Trop Med Hyg 2013;88(2):397–404.
17. The Merck Manual for Health Care Professionals, Eosinophilia. Available at: http://www.merckmanuals.com/professional/hematology_and_oncology/eosinophilic_disorders/eosinophilia.html. Accessed April 20, 2013.
18. Caumes E, Carriére J, Guermonprez G, et al. Dermatoses associated with travel to tropical countries: a prospective study of the diagnosis and management of 269 patients presenting to a tropical disease unit. Clin Infect Dis 1995;20:542–8.
19. Malhotra SK, Raj RT, Pal M. Cutaneous larva migrans in an unusual site. Dermatol Online J 2006;12(2):11.
20. Reported vectorborne and zoonotic diseases, U.S. Army and U.S. Navy, 2000-2011. MSMR 2012;19(10):15–6.
21. Jelinek T, Nothdruft HD, Rieder N, et al. Cutaneous myiasis: review of 13 cases in travelers returning from tropical countries. Int J Dermatol 1995;34:624–6.
22. Doherty JF, Grant AD, Bryceson AD. Fever as the presenting complaint of travelers returning from the tropics. Q J Med 1995;88:277–81.
23. MacLean J, Lalondi R, Ward B. Fever from the tropics. Travel Med Advisor 1994; 5:27.1–27.14.
24. O'Brien D, Tobin S, Brown GV, et al. Fever in returned travelers: review of hospital admissions for a 3-year period. Clin Infect Dis 2001;33:603–9.

Travel and Adventure Medicine Resources

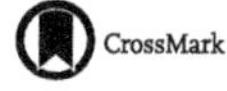

Christopher A. Sanford, MD, MPH, DTM&H[a,*], Paul S. Pottinger, MD, DTM&H, FIDSA[b]

KEYWORDS

• Travel medicine • Adventure medicine • Tropical medicine • Resources
• Professional associations • Continuing medical education • Online courses
• Textbooks

KEY POINTS

- It would behoove medical providers who provide pretravel consultations to join at least one travel or tropical medicine professional society, attend its annual meeting, and read its journal.
- Several textbooks on travel and adventure medicine are available, each of which has a particular focus (eg, travelers from high-income to low-income nations, tropical medicine, wilderness medicine, high-altitude medicine).
- A panoply of continuing medical education courses, both online and in person, are available; given the ever-changing nature of travel medicine, remaining current with these is a high priority.
- Practitioners can further their travel and tropical medicine skills by completing a degree course in tropical medicine; these are available in both low- and high-income nations.
- Several travel medicine applications are available, including the Centers for Disease Control and Prevention's *Health Information for International Travelers* (the Yellow Book.)

PROFESSIONAL ASSOCIATIONS AND SOCIETIES

There are numerous organizations dedicated to various aspects of tropical medicine, travel medicine, wilderness medicine, and particular specialties therein. Most publish journals and hold annual meetings.

- The International Society of Travel Medicine (ISTM) comprises more than 3200 medical providers and others with an interest in travel medicine in more than 90 countries. Members receive a subscription to the *Journal of Travel Medicine*; biennial 5-day conferences offer presentations on a wide variety of topics salient to traveler's health.[1]

[a] Family Medicine, Global Health, University of Washington, Box 358732, Seattle, WA 98125, USA; [b] Division of Allergy and Infectious Diseases, Department of Medicine, University of Washington, 1959 NE Pacific Street, Box 356130, Seattle, WA 98195, USA
* Corresponding author.
E-mail address: casanfo@uw.edu

Med Clin N Am 100 (2016) 411–416
http://dx.doi.org/10.1016/j.mcna.2015.09.004 medical.theclinics.com
0025-7125/16/$ – see front matter

- The American Society of Tropical Medicine and Hygiene (ASTMH) is a "worldwide organization of scientists, clinicians and program professionals" that was founded in 1903. Most of the Society's activities are in research, but there is a Clinical Group (American Committee on Clinical Tropical Medicine and Travelers' Health).[2]
- The UK-based Royal Society of Tropical Medicine and Hygiene (RSTMH) has clinician and researcher members in more than 130 countries. RSTMH fellows are charged with improving global health care "by facilitating training, education and the exchange of information."[3]
- The Wilderness Medical Society, founded in 1983, is focused on outdoor activities, including mountaineering. It publishes a journal, *Wilderness and Environmental Medicine*, and offers a variety of training opportunities, including a Diploma in Mountain Medicine.[4]
- Divers Alert Network (DAN) is a dive safety association. An excellent source of information regarding dive medicine, it provides consultative services and formal training. This association also sells reasonably priced insurance for emergency medical assistance and transportation in case of illness or injury while traveling.[5]
- International Society for Mountain Medicine was founded in 1985, with a goal of disseminating and developing high-quality information on mountain medicine. It publishes a quarterly journal, *High Altitude Medicine & Biology*.[6]
- The International Association for Medical Assistance to Travelers (IAMAT) is a Canada-based nonprofit that provides a list of approved clinics and English-speaking physicians around the world.[7] Given the wide variety of quality of medical care throughout middle- and low-income nations, travelers find this listing a useful resource.

CONTINUING MEDICAL EDUCATION COURSES

- Every 2 years, the University of Washington hosts a 2-and-a-half day conference on travel medicine for medical providers. Plenary presentations address immunizations, malaria, traveler's diarrhea, high-altitude medicine, and other topics salient to traveler's health. Information on this course is obtainable at the University of Washington's continuing medical education (CME) Web site.[8]
- The Harvard Humanitarian Institute, an academic research center based at the Department of Global Health and Population at the Harvard T.H. Chan School of Public Health, sponsors a variety of workshops pertaining to humanitarian emergencies.[9]
- Wilderness Medicine is a CME organization that offers a variety of courses, for both CME and certification in wilderness medicine, in locations around the globe.[10]

ONLINE COURSES

- The Centers for Disease Control and Prevention (CDC) maintains a Web site with several courses on tropical medicine and travel health. These courses are available to the public at no charge.[11]
- Human immunodeficiency virus (HIV) Web Study, which consists of several case-based modules concerning care for those with HIV/AIDS, is available online without charge. This educational program is funded through Health Resources and Services Administration, US Department of Health and Human Services.[12]
- The University of Minnesota offers a series of 7 modules that comprise their Online Global Health Course. Completion of this course partially fulfills the

content requirement for the ASTMH CTropMed examination.[13] The Director of the Global Health Course is William M. Stauffer III.

PRINTED MANUALS AND TEXTBOOKS

- CDC's *Health Information for the International Traveler* (Oxford University Press), better known as the Yellow Book, is a comprehensive reference on pretravel medicine, including immunizations, malaria, and traveler's diarrhea. It is available online at no charge; a hard copy, which is available for purchase, is published every 2 years.[14]
- *The Travel and Tropical Medicine Manual* (Elsevier) is a pocket-sized manual for health care providers. Elaine Jong edited the first edition, published in 1987; the fifth edition, edited by Christopher Sanford, Paul Pottinger, and Elaine Jong, will be published in 2016.
- *Tropical Infectious Diseases: Principles, Pathogens, and Practice* (Saunders), edited by Richard L. Guerrant, David H. Walker, and Peter F. Weller, is a comprehensive guide to tropical infections, with discussion of pathophysiology. The third edition was published in 2011.
- *Travel Medicine* (Elsevier), edited by Jay S. Keystone, Phyllis Kozarsky, David O. Freedman, Hans D. Nothdurft, and Bradley A. Connor, is a comprehensive text on the care of travelers to low-resource destinations. The third edition was published in 2012.
- *Hunter's Tropical Medicine and Emerging Infectious Disease* (9th edition, 2012) (Elsevier), edited by Alan J. Magill, Edward T. Ryan, David Hill, and Tom Solomon, provides a welcome balance of pathophysiology and pragmatic information for clinicians. Its lead editor, Dr Alan J. Magill, formerly a colonel in the US Army, was Director of the Malaria Program for the Bill and Melinda Gates Foundation at the time of his death in 2015.
- The *Oxford Handbook of Tropical Medicine* (Oxford University Press) is a "flexibound" handbook for clinicians in low-resource settings; it includes protocols developed by the World Health Organization. The fourth edition, edited by Robert Davidson, Andrew Brent, and Anna Seale, was published in 2014.
- The pre-eminent text on wilderness medicine is *Wilderness Medicine* (Mosby), edited by Paul S. Auerbach, a humungous (10.6 lbs) tome; its sixth edition was published in 2011.
- A superb case-based textbook of tropical medicine is *Clinical Cases in Tropical Medicine*, by Camilla Rothe (Elsevier 2015).
- *The Sanford Guide* is a high-quality pocket-sized reference for prescribing antibiotics, antivirals, antifungals, and antiparasitics. It is updated annually by a panel of experts.[15]

COURSES IN TROPICAL MEDICINE

Many clinicians who seek further training in tropical medicine will pursue a short course leading to a degree, e.g., a DTM&H (Diploma in Tropical Medicine & Hygiene).

- For clinicians with an interest in clinical work in Africa, the 3-month East African Diploma in Tropical Medicine and Hygiene provides an excellent overview of clinical tropical medicine. Hosted half in Tanzania, half in Uganda, each class of 60 to 70 students comprises physicians from Africa and from the Global North. This course is sponsored by a 5-institution consortium: Johns Hopkins University, Kilimanjaro Christian Medical University College (Moshi, Tanzania), the

London School of Hygiene and Tropical Medicine, Makerere University (Kampala, Uganda), and the University of Washington. The degree-granting entity is the London School of Hygiene and Tropical Medicine.[16]

- Another excellent clinical course is the 9-week Gorgas Course in Clinical Tropical Medicine.[17] This course, which is based in Lima, Peru, is sponsored jointly by the University of Alabama, Birmingham (UAB), and Universidad Peruaña Cayetano Heredia (UPCH). The UAB and UPCH directors of the Gorgas Course are German Henostroza and Eduardo Gotuzzo, respectively.
- Other courses are available in Bangkok, Berlin, London, Liverpool, and elsewhere; a full listing of Approved Diploma Courses in CTropMed is posted at the ASTMH Web site.[2]

FELLOWSHIPS

- Numerous research training fellowships are available. The National Institutes of Health–sponsored Fogarty Fellowships in Global Health are unsurpassed in terms of mentorship and training experience.[18]
- There are a rapidly growing number of clinical global health fellowships available to physicians. For example, the University of Washington's Department of Family Medicine Global Health Fellowship is targeted toward early-career family medicine physicians. More details regarding this 1-year fellowship are available at its Web site.[19]
- The University of Washington Department of Global Health also offers a variety of clinical and research fellowship opportunities for physicians in other specialties, including Internal Medicine.[20]
- There are a small number of wilderness medicine fellowships in the United States. The first, at Stanford University, California, was founded in 2003; this 1-year program accepts physicians who are board-certified or board-eligible in emergency medicine.[21] A full listing of wilderness medicine fellowships in the United States is available at the Web site of the Emergency Medicine Residents' Association.[22]

E-MAIL LISTSERVS

- ProMED (Program for Monitoring Emerging Diseases)-mail, established in 1994, is an Internet-based reporting system on "outbreaks of infectious diseases and acute exposures to toxins that affect human health, including those in animals and in plants grown for food or animal feed."[23] After signing up, an average of several e-mails detailing outbreaks and exposures will appear in your e-mail in-box daily. Alternatively, a weekly e-mail digest is available. All reports are vetted through a discerning moderator. The current editor is infectious disease specialist Lawrence C. Madoff, University of Massachusetts Medical School, Worcester. There is no charge to receive the e-mails; those who do may make contributions.

CERTIFICATES OF EXPERTISE

- There is no board certification in travel or tropical medicine; the closest approximation is the ASTMH Certificate of Knowledge (CTropMed). The examination leading to this certificate is now offered biennially. Requirements for sitting for the examination are listed at the ASTMH Web site.[24]
- A more limited examination, covering pretravel medicine only, is given annually by ISTM.[1] Those who pass this examination receive a Certificate in Travel Health.

A mandatory maintenance process, with retesting every 10 years, is required to keep the certification current.

INFORMATION ON CRIME, SECURITY, TERRORISM

- The US Department of State maintains an online list of statements on safety and security for every country in the world. In addition, this site lists Travel Alerts and Travel Warnings for selected nations; these are updated regularly.[25]

SUBSCRIPTION SERVICE

- For an annual fee, Shoreland Travax provides detailed country-specific information to health care providers. Of particular benefit are the detailed malaria and yellow fever maps that are provided as part of this service.[26]

APPLICATIONS

- The 2016 CDC *Health Information for International Travelers* (the Yellow Book) is available as an application (app); it can be accessed online as well as via the iTunes and GooglePlay app stores.
- The Shoreland Travax Web site can be browsed in a tablet environment.[24]
- The Sanford Guide app is a high-quality reference for prescribing antibiotics, antivirals, antifungals, and antiparasitics.[27]

REFERENCES

1. Available at: http://www.istm.org/index.asp. Accessed May 3, 2015.
2. Available at: https://www.astmh.org//AM/Template.cfm?Section=Home1. Accessed May 3, 2015.
3. Available at: https://rstmh.org/. Accessed May 3, 2015.
4. Available at: http://www.wms.org/. Accessed May 3, 2015.
5. Available at: http://www.diversalertnetwork.org/. Accessed May 3, 2015.
6. Available at: http://ismm.org/. Accessed July 30, 2015.
7. Available at: https://www.iamat.org/. Accessed May 3, 2015.
8. Available at: https://uw.cloud-cme.com/Ap2.aspx. Accessed May 3, 2015.
9. Available at: http://hhi.harvard.edu/. Accessed May 3, 2015.
10. Available at: http://www.wilderness-medicine.com/. Accessed July 30, 2015.
11. Available at: http://wwwnc.cdc.gov/travel/page/ce-courses-training. Accessed May 3, 2015.
12. Available at: http://www.hivwebstudy.org/. Accessed May 3, 2015.
13. Available at: http://www.globalhealth.umn.edu/education/online-global-health-course/. Accessed May 3, 2015.
14. Available at: http://wwwnc.cdc.gov/travel/page/yellowbook-home-2014. Accessed May 3, 2015.
15. Available at: http://www.sanfordguide.com/. Accessed July 30, 2015.
16. Available at: https://www.lshtm.ac.uk/study/cpd/eadtmh.html. Accessed May 3, 2015.
17. Available at: http://www.uab.edu/medicine/gorgas/. Accessed July 30, 2015.
18. Available at: http://www.fic.nih.gov/Programs/pages/scholars-fellows-global-health.aspx. Accessed July 30, 2015.
19. Available at: http://depts.washington.edu/fammed/residency/fellowships/global-health. Accessed May 3, 2015.
20. Available at: http://globalhealth.washington.edu/. Accessed July 30, 2015.

21. Available at: http://emed.stanford.edu/fellowships/wilderness.html. Accessed May 3, 2015.
22. Available at: http://www.emra.org/match/wilderness-medicine-fellowships/. Accessed May 3, 2015.
23. Available at: http://www.promedmail.org/. Accessed May 3, 2015.
24. Available at: http://www.astmh.org/Certification_Program/6521.htm. Accessed May 3, 2015.
25. Available at: www.state.gov. Accessed May 3, 2015.
26. Available at: http://www.shoreland.com/. Accessed May 3, 2015.
27. Available at: https://store.sanfordguide.com/storefront.aspx. Accessed July 30, 2015.

Index

Note: Page numbers of article titles are in **boldface** type.

Med Clin N Am 100 (2016) 417–433
http://dx.doi.org/10.1016/S0025-7125(16)00020-1 medical.theclinics.com

C

I

L

M

N

O

P

Q

R

S

U

Y

Z